Body Thoughts

Body Thoughts

Andrew J. Strathern

Ann Arbor
THE UNIVERSITY OF MICHIGAN PRESS

1999   1998   1997   4   3   2

A CIP catalog record for this book is available from the British Library

Library of Congress Cataloging-in-Publication Data

Strathern, Andrew.
    Body thoughts / Andrew J. Strathern.
       p.   cm.
    Includes bibliographical references (p.   ) and index.
    ISBN 0-472-09580-3 (hardcover : alk. paper). — ISBN 0-472-06580-7
 (pbk. : alk. paper)
    1. Body, Human—Social aspects.   2. Mind and body.   3. Ethnology—
 Melanesia.   4. Ethnology.   I. Title.
 GN298.S77   1996
    306.4—dc20   96-16550
                                                                 CIP

116974

Acknowledgments

In 1987, when I came to the University of Pittsburgh, I decided to begin teaching medical anthropology. My interest in this branch of anthropology grew initially out of my experiences during fieldwork for many years in Papua New Guinea and soon broadened into general questions of mind-body relations. Subsequently, I added a course on the anthropology of the body, and from this in turn came, in 1992, the idea for the present book. For friendly help in getting the original short proposal accepted by the University of Michigan Press, I wish to thank in particular Joyce Harrison (now with the University of South Carolina Press) and Professors Roy Rappaport and Raymond Kelly of the University of Michigan. Preparation of the book itself has been in various ways facilitated by Thomas Mullane, Kata Chillag, David Hudgens, and Abby Margolis, who have (by courtesy of the Dean's Office, Faculty of Arts and Sciences) worked for me successively as graduate student assistants at the University of Pittsburgh. The final version of the manuscript has benefited also from discussions in my Anthropology of the Body class in the fall of 1994, in which Jill Thomas Grannan, Satsuki Kawano, Joan Leach, Abby Margolis, Lisa Murphy, Tamiko Noll, Jo Recht, and John Traphagan took part. For discussions on the Duna materials I acknowledge the input of Dr. Gabriele Stürzenhofecker; and for views on the theme of chapter 7, I am indebted to Dr. Caryle Glosser and also to participants at the 1994 ASA conference, "Questions of Consciousness," held in St. Andrew's, Scotland. A version of this chapter is also published by Routledge in the ASA series of monographs edited by Anthony Cohen and Nigel Rapport, 1995. I thank also Patty Zogran, as usual, for her indefatigable work in typing and checking manuscript drafts and Dr. Pamela Stewart for help with final proofreading and indexing.

The completed manuscript itself also received a most perceptive review from the anonymous reader for the University of Michigan

Press. Indeed, in contradistinction to my experience on many other occasions, I found myself in close agreement with the reader's suggestions and lists of the book's shortcomings. I have tried briefly to respond to many of these comments but, regretfully, had to recognize that to meet all of them properly would mean prolonging the enterprise unduly. I wish to acknowledge here, however, some of the gaps in my exposition: feminist theorizing on and the efflorescence of an interest in "the body"; the work of Foucault, particularly his *History of Sexuality*, and sexuality in general; a proper appreciation and critique of Freud and Lacan, rather than my passing references here; and a full discussion of theories of magic from Hubert and Mauss through Malinowski, Leach, and Tambiah. Answering to the call of such topics properly would have meant, I fear, the addition of four more chapters, and this did not seem practicable (some are dealt with in Chris Shilling's book *The Body and Social Theory*). I therefore have committed the book to publication, while recognizing fully that its topic is almost indefinitely capable of expansion and any closure in the treatment of it is purely pragmatic and provisional.

Contents

Introduction

This book takes its inspiration from an essay that quickly established itself as a classic in its field: "The Mindful Body" by Margaret Lock and Nancy Scheper-Hughes (1987). My concern is to push the implications of that essay into ethnographic and topical areas, in which it can serve to re-illuminate issues to do with concepts of health and illness, personhood, and agency and with processes of change in sociocultural systems. Philosophical, historical, anthropological, and linguistic threads have to be woven together to make such a study.

In Western intellectual discourse discussion of the problems raised by Lock and Scheper-Hughes has often cited the work and influence of the French philosopher René Descartes, via his postulate of the absolute difference in kind between the soul (or "mind," but see below on this equation) and the body. While this is an advantageous perspective from the point of view of European intellectual history and therefore is also important as a means of understanding how scholars working within the various European traditions have themselves approached the concepts of a range of world cultures, it is necessary to recognize that in other ways starting from the Cartesian paradigm is arbitrary, both historically and cross-culturally. Indeed, the major reason for beginning differently is precisely that it can enable us to reject the Cartesian view, for European cultures as well as for many others across the globe.

Such a purpose in fact underlay Lock and Scheper-Hughes's enterprise also. Their concern was to retheorize mind-body relations in such a way as to highlight the concept of the body itself. This strategic tack has been followed by many others subsequently, to the extent that the term *embodiment* has reached the status of a major concept in cultural analysis (e.g., Csordas 1990). Yet, as both the term *embodiment* and Lock and Scheper-Hughes's own title indicate, it is not enough to switch from one side of the Cartesian dichotomy (i.e., mind) to the other (i.e., body) while leaving unquestioned the dichotomy itself. It is precisely the form of this dichotomy that has been contested and replaced implicitly or explicitly with concepts that stress crossover or interpenetration of putative mental and bodily characteristics, adding up to various forms of totality that express ideas similar to those encapsulated in earlier sociological terms such as *the individual* or *the person*. What, therefore, is gained by the use of a new terminology in which *embodiment* becomes central? It is simply that by this means we are reminded forcibly of a basic and ramifying feature of the human condition. Terms such as *individual* or *person* tend to have an abstract ring or reference, belonging to political and social philosophies that have to do with rights, identities, and tendencies of will or self-definition that are psychologically or legally based. *Embodiment,* by contrast, reminds us of the concrete, the here-and-now presence of people to one another, and the full complement of senses and feelings through which they communicate with one another (see Seremetakis 1994).

In the spirit of holism, which they have restimulated in social thinking, Lock and Scheper-Hughes begin "from an assumption of the body as simultaneously a physical and symbolic artifact, as both naturally and culturally produced, and as securely anchored in a particular historical moment" (1987, 7). We have to consider here what is meant by "simultaneously." Essentially, they are arguing that the body is a discrete entity that nevertheless carries separate meanings and aspects. It therefore becomes of interest to know not only what these separate aspects are but also, and perhaps more crucially, how they are related to or influence one another. They themselves distinguish "three bodies," by which they mean three semantic realms of representation and practice that use the image of the physical body as their locus of reference. The three bodies are the individual body, or the experiencing body in the phenomenological sense; the social body, in the sense used earlier by Mary Douglas, referring to the use of body imagery as a means of picturing social relations; and the "body politic," referring to the regulation of physical bodies by political and legal means (1987, 7–8).

It is clear that their list can be expanded or further compressed in accordance with heuristic needs. The social body overlaps with the political in a symbolic sense, since society always has coercive and therefore politicolegal aspects, and the practical effects of influence are always felt ultimately by the experiencing body of the individual. Skin tattoos, for example, are felt or experienced in a certain way; they may represent social values; and they may be restricted to, or enjoined on, a certain social class or category (see Gell 1993). Moreover, the body is "mindful" at all three of these levels, and there can be support, as well as interference, between them.

But what is meant by saying that the body is mindful? The statement appears to be a paralogism if we think along Cartesian lines. Certainly, we can interpret it as suggesting that the mind influences the body, but this would be to reinstitute the Cartesian dichotomy. Rather, what is being asserted here is that the basic concepts of reality that we have been accustomed to working with, especially in Western-style biomedicine, must be rethought. Since Descartes considered that the soul/mind had no physical extension (*res non extensa*) yet possessed the capacity to think (*res cogitans*) while the body had physical extension but no capacity to think, it is evident that he set up a realm of the physical, or material, that could be apprehended objectively as a "thing" and studied by the transcendental capacities of the soul/mind. The latter, however, remains mysterious in his usage, since it cannot be directly observed. Only the physical, in this sense, becomes both real and observable and thus becomes also the proper provenance of science. Observable reality becomes purely material, and hence there is a stress on the proximate material causes of things, including conditions of sickness. Such a mode of thought is much older than Descartes, of course. Lock and Scheper-Hughes cite the Greek Hippocratic tradition of medicine and the work of the philosopher Aristotle as belonging to the materialist persuasion with regard to sickness and the "soul" (*psūchē*). Descartes's arrangement of concepts, however, was quite different from Aristotle's. Whereas Aristotle concretized the soul (in line with earlier forms of Greek popular thought [see Onians 1954; Padel 1992]), Descartes preserved the soul for theology and the body for science (Lock and Scheper-Hughes 1987, 9), thus neatly keeping a foot in both camps in accordance with his own position as a Catholic. As biology and biomedicine developed, they tended, therefore, to leave out the mental aspect of somatic states.

A problem was thereby created for the understanding of phenomena classified as "mental illness." Such phenomena could not be studied directly if they were "mental." Yet they were accompanied by bodily states that were indubitably "there." The conundrum of mental illness is, in fact, simply an artifact of what we may call the Cartesian compromise between the impulses toward religion and science. Once we recognize that there is a mental component in all bodily states and, conversely, a physical component in all mental states, the boundary between mental and other illnesses disappears. Here, then, is a benefit to be derived from the idea of the mindful body.

As Genevieve Lloyd (1984) has argued, there is also an implicit gender component in European philosophical thought regarding the mind and the body. "Mind" has sometimes been equated with the male sphere of reason and culture and "body" with the female sphere of emotions and nature, the former clearly represented as superior to the latter (see also MacCormack and Strathern 1980; Schiebinger 1993). Such a conflation of categories is unlikely to have resulted purely from the thoughts of philosophers themselves. Rather, it is likely to have derived from prevailing popular or religious ideologies that found their way into the thoughts of philosophers either consciously or unconsciously. Descartes himself makes no such explicit correlations, but his extreme separation of the soul from the body made it possible not only to isolate the sphere of reason and the intellect from the sphere of practical, embodied life but also to exaggerate the male-female dichotomy that was grafted onto this dichotomy of mind and body. It is important to note at once that this act of ideological grafting is one that is culturally specific and not necessarily universal, although it may have widespread analogies in other cultures. The effect, however, of such an ideological structure of thought can still be observed in popular Euro-American culture, in which, for example, the expression of emotions may be seen as appropriate only to females (and then not always), while males are represented as rational and are expected to maintain "a stiff upper lip" (Lutz 1988).

Descartes, according to Lloyd, drew some of his inspiration from Plato, whose views also idealized pure and rarefied thought as the source of true knowledge (*epistēmē*) (Lloyd 1984, 47). This kind of theory of knowledge also tends to unite religion and science. Descartes, for example, considered that the intellect is the part that unites man to God, although God is supposed to have created both mind (or soul) and body "in his own image" (see Hanson 1979). By another twist, emptying the body of all vestiges of the soul freed scientists to examine the body physically as a thing, thus facilitating the growth of experimental biology. By the same token, however, Descartes's dichotomy might imply a ban on any attempt to "investigate" the soul by empirical methods.

Descartes's own enterprise was a complex one, selectively cited in later times as a justification for further enterprises of a theological, philosophical, or scientific kind. His work became in the anthropological sense a founding charter for biomedical practice and theory. At the same time it preserved a hierarchy of mind over matter that was essentially theocentric. His idea that the soul does not have a physical extension saves the concept of the soul from any attempts to study it by physical means and thus makes it a secure object for contemplation by thought alone. Where he derived this notion from is perhaps hard to say, since in most religious systems the soul is given some physical existence, however ethereal. Similarly, his ambiguous conflation of soul with mind is one that cannot be exactly paralleled in Germanic and English-speaking traditions of thought but belongs, instead, to the French language and its apparent identification of *âme* (from Latin *anima*) with *esprit* (from Latin *spiritus*) (see, however, Parkin 1985, 149). Commentators who ignore differences of meaning in this semantic arena between different European languages run the risk of blurring the issues involved.

A problem for Descartes, as for all Cartesianists subsequently, is how to account for the intermingling of mind and body, given their absolute difference and separation. In some fashion Descartes gave the soul/mind an ethnolocation within the head, since he considered that the point of interaction between soul and body was the pineal gland. This small gesture toward physicalization could have led to a more thoroughgoing recognition or investigation of these links as is now conducted under the rubric, for example, of psychoneuroimmunology, but for Descartes the gesture was sufficient. He does not seem to have been interested in following it up, perhaps for the good reason that to do so would have undermined his whole a priori position.

In medical anthropology Descartes has become negatively significant, for example, in Lock and Scheper-Hughes's narrative, as the source for the mechanistic-materialistic background to biomedicine. Whether this corresponds historically to his own exact aims is another matter. It is with the intervening trajectory of history that medical anthropologists have had to contend and, in the course of doing so, to recreate the anthropology of the body along the lines argued for by

Lock and Scheper-Hughes. In a collection entitled *Giving the Body Its Due* Albert A. Johnstone has taken up the cause by reentering the correspondence between Descartes and Princess Elizabeth of Bohemia (Johnstone 1992, 16 ff.). Johnstone further equates the soul with the "self," a move that is potentially confusing although it may be necessary for his argument. His main purpose, however, is to argue that Elizabeth was right in her questions to Descartes and that if he had answered them properly, he would have remained more consistent with his own rational epistemic values. Johnstone's aim is thus to turn Descartes upside down. Elizabeth asked Descartes how the soul can act on the body, since it lacks the properties by which one body acts on another. She further pointed out that bodily matters such as emotions do apparently affect the soul's ability to engage in clear reflections. The basis of her question is thus her own introspection. In reply Descartes suggested that the union of body and soul accounts for the imagination and thus the effect of troubling thoughts on the soul itself. But this presupposes exactly what Elizabeth was questioning. She was, in fact, suggesting that emotions or feelings have an effect on the soul, perhaps also alluding to earlier views about the divided soul (Lloyd 1984, 18). It was precisely this view that Descartes's own scheme was designed to replace, yet his answers to Elizabeth's objections were not very convincing. Johnstone goes on to argue that the "felt body" is a phenomenological basis for the knowledge of oneself as a being that exists and that this knowledge is different from Descartes's cogito principle. Probably this is why Johnstone equates soul with self. In fact, he shifts here from Descartes's "language game" to his own. Descartes's soul is not the self as represented in phenomenological philosophy. It is more like a portion or reflection of the divine intellect, an idea that has no place in phenomenology as such.

Given, however, that Johnstone wishes essentially to subvert Descartes's concepts with his own and to base this move on the idea of the felt body, his argument is obviously important for us here. Negating the technical arguments of Sartre and Merleau-Ponty on this topic (Johnstone 1992, 24–25), he turns to his own introspection, as Elizabeth of Bohemia also seems to have done, believing that this can be purified from its cultural tinges (26), a proposition that an anthropologist would find unnecessary as well as doubtful, since the "inside" that one "looks into" is also culturally constructed. He notes that Descartes located some feelings, such as joy and anger, within the soul and not in the body (a curious fact in itself, given Descartes's overall aim of preserving a realm of pure intellect). In Descartes's own scheme, then, it is hard to see how such feelings would relate to the body. Yet, as Johnstone points out, we experience emotions in the body: "one invariably finds some modification of one's felt body, that same body in which are located one's pains, one's hunger, and one's feeling of warmth" (28). In making this observation, Johnstone is certainly following in the footsteps of observational physiologists (e.g., Cannon 1932), and his argument is presumably right in terms of his own experience also. He is probably on less strong ground when he rejects conclusions from an experimental finding that the emotional tenor of a social occasion influenced subjects injected with epinephrine (a stimulant) into reporting either anger or euphoria (30). Johnstone opposes this interpretation of the experiment, since it would suggest that the experience of emotions is contextualized by events outside of the introspective self and thus that there is a social or cultural dimension to the experience. Again, for the anthropologist such a finding poses no threat; indeed it is an essential starting point. What we call "emotions" are culturally laden concepts *as well as* deeply felt bodily states. There is here a conjunction of the social and the personal, which it is part of our stock-in-trade to study (see Battaglia 1995).

With the introduction of these social or cultural elements I will now turn back from philosophy to the stream of anthropological theorizing about the body, but the philosophical background must always be kept in mind as relevant. This conjunction between anthropology and philosophy is marked well also by Margaret Lock in her later important survey article, "Cultivating the Body: Anthropology and Epistemologies of Bodily Practice and Knowledge" (1993). Lock's article provides a bibliographic background to the particular project on which I embark here. She discusses the history of approaches to the social and cultural construction of the body/bodies in anthropological analyses, especially in medical anthropology (see also Featherstone, Hepworth, and Turner 1991). One point she makes, however, is especially relevant: that an anthropology of the body must include a theory of the emotions, and the first step toward such a theory is to recognize how arbitrary the Cartesian separation between "reason" and "emotion" is. Citing the work of the medical anthropologist Gilbert Lewis (1980) and the cultural anthropologist Michelle Rosaldo (1984), she indicates that "emotions inevitably involve both meaning and feeling" and "thus emotions cannot simply be captured as either cognitive judgements or visceral reactions" (Lock 1993, 139). Hence Rosaldo's term *embodied thought*, which has given rise to my title here, *Body Thoughts*. Lock's article can be read in conjunction both with this introduction and with my conclusions in chapter 8. Yet it is interesting to add to the well-based constructivism of her approach evidence from recent studies of the human brain itself, which indicate that the neural pathways of the brain implicate together what we label as emotions and rational thought, in particular via the amygdala. Work by Antonio Damasio (1994) has been prominent here, and Damasio has explicitly undertaken to argue that Descartes was wrong to associate reason with the brain and emotion with the body, since the body itself, self-perceived in the brain, is actually the basis of what we experience as mind (on neural nets, see also Kosslyn and Koenig 1992). It is interesting to realize that these latest findings by neurophysiologists would be found unsurprising by many peoples around the world who know nothing about neurophysiology but in whose own cultural concepts emotion and reason are closely linked (e.g., Wikan 1990, on Bali).

With this point in mind I now begin to retrace the steps of constructivist theorists of the body, starting with Marcel Mauss and moving to Mary Douglas.

Chapter 1

The Social Body: Mauss
to Douglas

In two boldly constructed works the British social anthropologist Mary Douglas drew together many trends implicit in the writings of French authors, from Emile Durkheim and his nephew Marcel Mauss onward (see Fournier 1994, 25–26), in order to develop her own synthesis of ideas regarding the body, pollution, taboos, social categories, and the sources of ritual symbolism (Douglas 1970, [1966] 1984). Douglas has been a true Durkheimian in her basic orientations within anthropology. She takes seriously the proposition that categories of thought are socially derived and that their explanation is to be sought in elucidating the social conditions from which they spring. If we accept this proposition, greatly contested as it has been, it follows that categorizations that surround and define the body must have a social origin. To argue this is the reverse of the familiar proposition that the body has sometimes been taken, in an organic analogy, as the image or model of society (hence phrases such as "the body politic"). Alternatively, without assigning causal priorities we can study how images of the body are mapped onto society and vice versa.

Durkheim was himself largely concerned with establishing an empirical study of social facts (treating them as "things" [*choses*]) and with arguing for the social origins of widespread phenomena such as religion (Durkheim [1912] 1968). Mauss was more concerned than Durkheim with the question of the body, and he preserved also a historical or evolutionary viewpoint within his writings. Two of his later works are particularly significant in relation to the body: his essays on "the notion of person" (1938) and on "the techniques of the body" (1935). Mauss himself does not appear to have synthesized these two separate sketches of the topics involved, although Csordas (1990), using the concept of embodiment, has subsequently attempted an exer-

9

cise along such lines. The essay on the body is a straightforward demonstration of the effect of social rules and conditioning on the physical bodies of individuals, a theme that resonates most clearly with the subsequent work of Michel Foucault (e.g., Foucault 1979). It fits also with the detailed observations of other anthropologists, for example, Malinowski's remark that sexual practices among the Trobrianders of Papua New Guinea had their own specific form, and the same argument has fed into the work of Pierre Bourdieu and Paul Connerton on memory and social conditioning (see chap. 2). This piece by Mauss therefore is clearly consonant with aspects of contemporary thinking about the body. Its referent is the physical body itself, as molded by society and culture.

The essay on the person, which has been more favored by commentators in the past, has a more indirect, but still important, relationship to the topic of the body as a site for the expression of social personhood or individuality. The issue of individuality is one that must be dealt with separately. Mauss takes an evolutionary standpoint, arguing that notions of individuality emerged only in the course of European history, out of earlier concepts of *"personnage"* (role or character) as well as the primordial concept of the self (*le "moi"*), which he acknowledged to be universal (Mauss 1985, 3; trans. W. D. Halls, in Carrithers et al. 1985). For the most part Mauss, in fact, concentrates on the idea of *personnage* in a range of preindustrial societies, linking this with the practice of assigning limited sets of names to people belonging to different clans. These names are seen by him as defining roles whose overall purpose is to act out "the prefigured totality of the life of the clan" (5). The individual appears only as the bearer and transmitter of one of these roles and of the ritual powers associated with them and achieved through spirit possession. *Personnage* becomes transmuted in Roman law into *persona,* a legal entity, to which, however, certain ritual masks (i.e., *persona* in the original sense) might belong. The legal reference of the term can be seen in the fact that slaves did not possess it: *servus non habet personam* (17).

Mauss goes on to argue that further alterations came about with Christianity, in which the legal concept of "persona" was transformed theoretically into a universal idea of the "human person." It is this Christian idea, it appears, that is sometimes used by subsequent writers to make a contrast between "Western" thought and that of tribal societies (see Burridge 1979). Finally, Mauss notes that the idea of the human person as a psychological being within society is a still later elaboration. In one of the abrupt transitions that characterize his wide-ranging work, he switches into discussion of the work of philosophers and credits Spinoza, Hume, Kant, and, finally, Fichte with developing a concept of the self (*moi*). This concept could function as the basis of consciousness, reason, and ethics and, hence, became the source of political philosophies such as were promulgated by Thomas Paine and fed into the Declaration of Independence of the first thirteen states of the United States of America. Glancingly, Mauss refers this development also to theorizing regarding the soul but gives only fleeting notice in this context to Descartes, awarding instead his accolade to Spinoza for pursuing the ethical dimension of discussion regarding the soul.

Here, as elsewhere, Mauss seems to move too swiftly over rough ground. He introduces an idea of the self as primordial only to abandon it and reemerge at the end of his discussion with the same idea now given an apparently new meaning. And he brings in the matter of the soul and its immortality only in the final part of his inquiry instead of asking whether it, too, has relevance for the definition of the self in all of the societies he surveys. Nevertheless, in broad terms his message is clear: ideas of the self and the person are socially constructed and vary historically, a process he tends to treat as progressive or evolutionary in some sense.

Nick Allen in his commentary on Mauss's essay points out that we need not overstress this evolutionary thread in Mauss's thought (Allen 1985, 27–29) but that Mauss's concern, whether evolutionary in any unilineal sense or otherwise, was with concepts as they operated in the "legal and moral spheres" (*droit et morale*) (29) and also as parts of social totalities for which Mauss was building up a model. Allen also notes that this model may have been in a sense a mirage, since its full equivalent in ethnographic fact may not be found (41). For our purposes here it is more important to seek out the analytical connections between Mauss's discussions of the person and of bodily techniques. The linking concept, in fact, is found in the latter essay, in which he writes (as translated by Ben Brewster [Mauss 1979, 101]) on the term *habitus*, after discoursing on different patterns of swimming, marching, and running:

> Hence I have had this notion of the social nature of the *habitus* for many years. Please note that I use the Latin word—it should be

understood in France—*habitus*. The word translates infinitely better than *habitude* (habit or custom), the "exis" [should be *hexis*], the
"acquired ability" and "faculty" of Aristotle (who was a psychologist). It does not designate those metaphysical *habitudes*, that mysterious "memory."

Mauss attributes variations in *habitus* in this sense to the "work of
collective and individual practical reason" rather than to "merely the
soul and its repetitive faculties" (ibid.). That is, he sees *habitus* as historically variable rather than universal—in other words, as the embodiment of cultural difference encoded in education. It is in a way remarkable that he introduces the concept in this way without reference to
concepts of person/self, since one of the obvious ways in which these
latter are constructed is precisely in terms of bodily *habitus*. Ideas of this
kind were not peculiar to Mauss or to French traditions of thought
either, since they are to be found also in the writings of the German ethnologist Richard Thurnwald in his book *Banaro Society*, first published
in 1916:

> The institutions of the social organization dominate the individ-
> ual to such a degree that his actions become almost automatic and
> are generally no more considered than is his gait or the fingers of a
> good piano player. This automatization of our thinking and the
> prearrangement of our personal behavior by formalities saves
> energies and facilitates the conscious process in the reciprocal rela-
> tions. (Thurnwald 1916, 390)

This quotation also gives us one clue why Mauss himself did not
link *habitus* with *personne*. *Habitus* calls to mind the unconscious and
personne the conscious aspects of ourselves, and Mauss was interested
in tracing the history of ideas about consciousness, among other things,
in his essay on the person. For a full theoretical perspective, however,
we need to juxtapose *habitus* with more consciously developed elements of personality, especially since Mauss insists that *habitus* is
learned, not natural, as in the traditional way of walking called *onioni*,
taught by Maori mothers to their daughters (Mauss 1979, 102). In this
example the teaching and learning are at first fully conscious. It is only
afterward that the learned pattern becomes an unconscious part of bodily routines.

The rest of Mauss's discussion is largely taken up with further examples of learned forms of *habitus*. There is, however, an elegant overall formulation that sums up his starting point and has become a starting point for others, such as Mary Douglas (1970):

> The body is man's first and most natural instrument. Or more accurately, not to speak of instruments, man's first and most natural technical object, and at the same time, technical means, is his body. (Mauss 1979, 104)

Mauss extends this fundamental observation into the sphere of theorizing about magic. Here he writes that "technical action, physical action, magico-religious action are confused for the actor" (1979, 103). Whether we say that there is "confusion" here or simply "fusion" is moot, but in any case it is the embodied, action-oriented aspect of magical techniques that is highlighted. Words and movements act out desired ends. In one example, from an old account of an Australian Aboriginal hunting ritual, a hunter carries a piece of magical rock crystal in his mouth and chants a formula as he climbs a tree in order to dislodge a possum that he is hunting. As Mauss points out, the magical action is also a part of a practical and concurrent bodily movement and contributes, in fact, to the efficacy of that movement. This embodied characteristic of magic is therefore central to our understanding of magic as a total practice.

Mauss's observations on bodily techniques therefore fan out in a number of directions relevant to the anthropology of the body overall, and I return to some of them in the next chapter. Here I move on to the work of Mary Douglas, which is predicated both on fundamental Durkheimian propositions that also permeate Mauss's work and, specifically, on the idea of the body as a natural symbol, similar to Mauss's picture of it as man's "first and most natural instrument."

It is in her second work on the theme of the body, *Natural Symbols* (1970) that Douglas most explicitly follows Mauss's pointers, albeit with her own twists. In other senses, however, *Purity and Danger* is both intellectually and chronologically prior and should be discussed first. The body as a natural symbol in fact appears early on in *Purity and Danger* (henceforth *PD*) but in an abstract, intellectualist way that is reminiscent also of Lévi-Strauss: "The body is a model which can stand for any kind of bounded system" (Douglas [1966] 1984, 115). The

Durkheimian movement of her thought is shown immediately after this quotation, when she writes that

> we cannot possibly interpret rituals concerning excreta, breast milk, saliva and the rest unless we are prepared to see in the body a symbol of society, and to see the powers and dangers credited to social structure reproduced in small on the human body. (ibid.)

Part of her reason for asserting this viewpoint is to oppose psychological reductionism, as Mauss also did, especially the version of psychology that compares the cultural practices of so-called primitive peoples with those of deviant individuals in European societies. An example of theorizing of this kind that she correctly ridicules is the idea that among primitive peoples the ego is weakly developed and infantile wishes are still expressed in adulthood, so that "archaic man retains the magic body of infancy" (117; quoting Norman O. Brown).

Douglas replaces this form of reductionism with her own Durkheimian brand of sociological determinism, when she argues that it is in the form of social practices and the symbolism of boundaries associated with these that the explanation of particular ideas about the body are to be found. She uses this standpoint in a good cause when criticizing psychological interpretations that depend on the equation "primitive man = child." For example, she argues that bodily symbols may be used in an adult and serious way to confront problems of separation and loss in social life, as in funeral rituals in which people as mourners first take onto their bodies forms of rubbish or dirt and then cleanse themselves (Douglas [1966] 1984, 121, 176–77, on the Nyakyusa people). Bodily exuviae may also be used as vehicles of political power, as when fluids from the corpse of a queen among the Lovedu people of the Drakensberg mountains in South Africa are used by the successor queen to control the weather by magical means (120). These are valid examples, although it is possible to argue along Freudian lines that all these practices, while owing their specific content to cultural traditions, may take their genesis from intrapsychic processes. Douglas's own purpose with these examples is to home in on one of her central problems: "Why should bodily margins be thought to be specially invested with power and danger?"

Her answer is that since the cultural concern (in the sense of sets of symbolic meanings) with such margins is variable, the causes of symbolism are to be found in society (i.e., processes and social relations realized in practice): we should proceed "from the known dangers of society to the known selection of bodily themes and try to recognize what appositeness is there." (Douglas [1966] 1984, 121)

It is worthwhile to notice here exactly what the focus is. It is on margins rather than total sets of ideas about the body and the person. We are thus exploring only a section of our overall topic but one that enables Douglas to pursue her sociological reasoning. Second, the thinking is purely sociocentric, focused on the standardized "social body." These two points are well-known and have been much canvassed. Third, however, perhaps the most interesting and productive part of Douglas's assertions lies in her recommendation that we look for concordances between social dangers and their bodily symbols. Concordance, appositeness: these are ideas that suggest matters of logical fit. But, if we wish to deepen the approach, we can also broaden the notion of appositeness, as I will do later. Let us first consider Douglas's own arguments and examples, expressed with her own crisp élan.

First, she develops a typology of social pollution: (1) "danger pressing on external boundaries"; (2) "danger from transgressing the internal lines of the system"; (3) "danger in the margins of the lines"; and (4) "danger from internal contradiction" (Douglas [1966] 1984, 122). The "danger" involved in all of these contexts is that of social breakdown (or social change, to view it from another perspective). With this definition it is clearly assumed that bodily symbolism is used ultimately to maintain the status quo. The argument is therefore functionalist although, again, we could quite easily twist it to point out that the same forms of symbolism can be used for the purposes of resistance, rebellion, or even revolution.

The examples Douglas chooses illustrate her concern with social rigidity versus fluidity. Her first example is the Coorg society of south India. Coorgs had a great fear of impurities entering their bodies, and this was related to their caste system, in which higher castes guarded against impurity from lower castes; yet there was a division of labor in which lower castes performed menial and polluting tasks on behalf of higher ones. The social order was seen as like a body, in which "the head [i.e., the higher castes] does the thinking and praying and the most despised parts [the lower castes] carry away the waste matter" (Douglas [1966] 1984, 123). The Coorgs' preoccupation with boundaries belongs to Douglas's category 2 but also, she suggests, to category 1,

since they were an isolated minority group within a wider society. She
implies that they were anxious to preserve their separation (whether it
was objectively threatened or not), as were the ancient Israelites, a
beleaguered people. "The threatened boundaries of their [the
Israelites'] body politic would be well mirrored in their care for the
integrity, unity, and purity of the physical body." (124) Paradoxically,
she herself notes that this care did not extend, in the Indian case, to
taboos on where and how people actually defecated (124). It is apparent that the ethnographic materials she cites raise more questions than
they answer. Another example that she throws in, that of the Yurok of
northern California (Klamath River), produces the same effect. Noting
that these people had many taboos regarding the mixing of fluids, especially sea and river water, she suggests that such taboos be seen against
the backdrop of the "fluid formlessness of their highly competitive
social life" (127). It is not clear here why in the Coorg case taboos
against inappropriate mixing should reflect rigidity while in the Yurok
case apparently similar rules should have been precipitated (by a contrary dialectic?) out of fluidity and formlessness.

Douglas is quite aware that many of her examples may not be fully
worked out. Her aim is to exemplify a theory and a method and to sum
up her conclusions in a pithy manner, as at the end of chapter 7: "rituals work upon the body politic through the symbolic medium of the
physical body." (Douglas [1966] 1984, 128) Here she suggests that rituals use the physical body in order to effect social operations, to make
statements about political structure. It is a valuable generalization and
one that surely resonates with, for example, the work of Victor
Turner—but, whereas Turner was *also* concerned with the psychophys-
iological level, Douglas has her eyes uncompromisingly fixed on "society" as such. A more phenomenological approach would attempt to
bring these two levels of society and the individual more closely
together.

Like Mauss, Douglas is interested in the moral dimension of acts,
and she raises the question of how ideas about bodily pollution may be
related to morals. Here she is on solid ethnographic ground. She goes
to the corpus of writings by Evans-Pritchard on the Nuer (one of her
favorite sources) and points out that, while the Nuer have rules and
ideas that express the dangers of incest and adultery in general, their
attitude to any particular case is not very disapproving. Their pollution
ideas serve to support the rules while deflecting immediate disap-

proval away from miscreants. Thus, adultery can be dangerous to the offended husband because of the pollution it causes: hence, he must be compensated and a sacrifice made by the adulterer. The adulterer himself is not at risk of becoming sick, it should be noted. Pollution ideas uphold the rules, but, if compensation is made, no further moral disapproval comes into play.

Douglas makes a further observation of a functionalist kind here and turns it into a general hypothesis. Some rules are supported by mystical sanctions, others are not. A Nuer son should respect his father yet, even if he fails to do so, he does not incur the mystical danger he would for neglecting to honor his parents-in-law. A father has economic sanctions he can bring to bear on his son, whereas in-laws cannot exercise control in this way; hence, Douglas argues, it is the *weaker* relationship that is buttressed by ideas of pollution. Her general hypothesis is that pollution beliefs come into play in areas of social structure in which clear-cut secular or material constraints do not operate. They thus act, in her view, as supplementary mechanisms of social control. Numerous ethnographic examples can be cited that fit with this hypothesis, including beliefs "that a woman will miscarry if she has committed adultery while pregnant" (Douglas [1966] 1984, 134), for instance, or an example from Papua New Guinea not given by Douglas, the Pangia people's idea that a woman who has committed adultery will have difficulty in giving birth unless and until she confesses to her adulteries (in one case known to me the woman confessed to sixteen separate acts with different men before her child was safely born). Ideas of this kind can also have ramifying results. For example, the Bemba people considered that pollution can be conveyed through fire, which is also a medium of cooking; hence, women were at great pains to renew their sources of fire periodically from neighbors who were considered ritually pure (138).

If we reexamine these and other examples Douglas gives, not so much from a functionalist (or antifunctionalist) standpoint but, rather, in pursuit of the mindful body, it is clear that her themes fit well with such a focus. The link between "pollution" (a physical concept in a sense) and "morals" shows exactly the conjunction of body and mind we would expect to find. Actions that are the product of will and intention have repercussions on the bodies of those involved, and the incidence of these repercussions tells us how the moral universe is structured. Equally, however, it reveals the ethnotheories of the people themselves about flows of substances and powers between persons. Why is it, for example, that for the Nuer an adulterous man is not at risk from the mystical influence of the woman's husband, while the husband himself *is* thought to be at risk? Clearly, in Nuer theory the flow of power (literally of confusion) runs from adulterer to husband, that is, from polluter to polluted, via the sexual organs of the woman. It is the one who is wronged who becomes sick, not the wrongdoer(s). This is an idea that chimes with some concepts of the Hagen people in Papua New Guinea regarding anger and sickness. Anger arises in a wronged person, and, through the action of ghosts on the person's *noman* ("mind"), it can cause sickness, which can then be cured only through revealing the cause of the anger and extracting compensation from the miscreant. The difference between the Nuer and the Hagen examples here is that, in the Nuer case, effects are held to flow automatically, while, in Hagen, the victim of wrongdoing must know the cause and experience resentment against it. In both cases, however, immoral acts cause sickness, and thus the body, by definition, becomes mindful. In addition, in Melanesian contexts, and perhaps African ones too, some ethnotheory of substances seems to be implicated as a kind of "chemistry." In the case of adultery, for example, it is the "semen out of place" that pollutes the woman's body and secondarily her husband's (through inappropriate mixing [see Héritier-Augé 1979, 1994]), thus causing sickness.

If we return now to Douglas's own work, we find that in her second book on the body, *Natural Symbols,* she has systematized her theories of social structure but never abandons her Durkheimian principles. In chapter 5 she argues that "the social body constrains the way the physical body is perceived" (Douglas 1970, 68). Thus, bodily control is an expression of social control (as Mauss argued, using the idea of *habitus*). In the original edition of her book she took the body itself as a "natural" basis for social symbolism, but in a later edition she admits that the physical body is already socially constructed and that its physiological constraints "could never give rise to the variety of symbolic structures based on it." (23).

In order to systematize her arguments Douglas introduces in this book her theory of grid and group. In societies in which "grid" (the presence of unbounded role networks) is stressed, the inner self comes to be a focus whereas, in those stressing "group" (bounded collectivity of one kind or another), outward necessities are more important than motivation. In my commentary here I am not concerned with the over-all grid/group theory other than to note that there should be correlations between grid/group patterns and ethnotheories of the body. In this context two of Douglas's discussions are of particular interest. In one she considers trance and possession, in another the presence or absence of ideas of menstrual pollution. With regard to trance she argues that trance states will be "feared as dangerous when the social dimension is highly structured but welcomed and even deliberately induced when this is not the case" (Douglas 1970, 74). If we see the body as a model of society and trance with possession as a breach of the body's boundaries, it does make sense to argue that such a breach may be considered more threatening in societies in which rigid control (i.e., defense of group boundaries) is important. Douglas's own example, however, shows the limitation of this line of reasoning. She notes that for the Nuer people trance is held to be dangerous, whereas for their neighbors, the Western Dinka, it is a blessing. Presumably, this should be a mark of greater rigidity in Nuer social structure. Yet for the Nuer also if a man is possessed permanently by a spirit he becomes a prophet, who thereafter occupies an abnormal, "wild" role, transcending the ordinary divisions between political groups. In colonial times (when Evans-Pritchard worked with the Nuer in what was then the Anglo-Egyptian Sudan) such prophets sometimes became foci of political resistance to the British. A similar potentiality lies in the role of the Flesh spearmasters among the Dinka and the leopard-skin priests among the Nuer themselves, who also appeal to the divinity Flesh as the source of their power. The appeal here does seem to be to the individual body of certain men as repositories of power that can transgress political divisions usually operative in society. The image of the divinity Flesh becomes a means of conceptualizing historical change. In this way we learn more from the Nuer/Dinka example than can be done by treating it as a flat case of synchronic structural comparison.

The argument regarding menstrual pollution also begins as a static comparison. Here Douglas takes two small-scale hunter-gatherer societies of Africa, the Mbuti and the Hadza. As with most such societies, social groupings in both cases are fluid. In theory, therefore, neither should show a concern for boundaries expressed in terms of pollution. The Mbuti conform: they have no pollution ideas. The Hadza men, however, show a fear of menstrual blood. Douglas correlates this not with social group but with gender boundaries. There is a marked division between the sexes among Hadza, and pollution fears reflect and maintain this division. Yet a Hadza husband is also expected to stress his tie to his wife by practicing a kind of "couvade" at the time of her menstrual seclusion. In Douglas's terms this reads like a way of supporting a potentially weak tie by means of mystical ideas. But, while the comparison between the Mbuti and the Hadza is thereby made and explained, further questions arise. Why do the Hadza have sexual separation? Is there gender hierarchy among them? What ethnotheory of the body and its substances explains the custom of menstrual couvade? How do gender representations alter over time? Are there—and this is a crucial general point—different gendered ideas of the body? The account Douglas gives of cargo cults among the Hadza indicates the importance of shifting again from a synchronic to a historical mode in pursuing the analysis (1970, chap. 9).

Sanday (1981, 92 ff.) has also argued that we need to take ecological variables into account. She notes that there is not only male fear of female menstrual pollution among the Hadza but also a strong consciousness of difference and antagonism between the sexes, which is at its height in dry times, "when camps are bigger and humans congregate near the few available sources of water" (93). She proposes to link the Hadza men's practices of hunting large game outside of their camps and gambling within them with the idea of "danger," which she claims is symbolized in fears of menstrual pollution. But this explanation lacks any way of showing the "appositeness" between the symbol and what it stands for that Mary Douglas called for. A simpler approach to explaining Hadza ideas would be via the analyses of "bride-service societies" made by Collier and Rosaldo (1981). They point out that there is potentially a good deal of sexual competition within or between hunter-gatherer bands and that a man has often a long struggle to secure a bride for himself. A concern with sexual segregation and concomitant fears of pollution would then be one way of handling or controlling such competition. Collier and Rosaldo have also argued that in these societies the interests of men and women diverge markedly with regard to marriage and sexual relations in general. Segregation and antagonism could therefore be expected, though not necessarily fears of pollution. Given the cultural existence of such fears, we can also easily understand why they should be more pronounced in the dry season camps, which bring more people together and therefore increase the likelihood of sexual competition and disputes arising out of it.

Overall, Mary Douglas is basically more interested in the social than in the physical body, since "the social body constrains the way the physical body is perceived." From a contemporary perspective, however, it is important always to remember that the social body *is* also the physical body, and vice versa. There may be several analytical frameworks for discussion, but the material body tends to be implicated in all of them. And the cultural theory of that body is the mechanism whereby the physical is linked to the social. It is also the piece that until recently tended to be missing from the ethnography of kinship and gender, for example. We do not need to suppose here that "the social" directly constrains "the physical," since both meet and are articulated in "the cultural"—i.e., the realm of attribution of meanings to events and processes. This point can be explored further by considering some of the literature on New Guinea societies that has been extensively canvassed since Douglas's two books were written.

Many, if not most, of the societies of the New Guinea Highlands are characterized by rules regarding menstrual dangers that act to keep the sexes spatially separated for definite periods of time. They are also characterized by gender hierarchy and the exercise of dominance by senior males. It is not hard to make a functional link between separation, hierarchy, and dominance and to perceive cultural ideas regarding menstruation as a form of ideology. From there it is only another short step to hitch the analysis onto what was in the 1970s a neo-Marxist wagon. In general, the main form of such analyses can be sustained but without a strict adherence to Marxist propositions as such (a solution that is unlikely to please either committed Marxists or committed deconstructionists [see M. Strathern 1988]). Yet, the problems of comparison and change remain. For example, some societies marked by at least a degree of gender domination do not appear to have shown great concern for menstrual dangers. Two cases are the Kuma of mid-Wahgi (Reay 1959; O'Hanlon 1989) and the Wiru of Pangia (Strathern 1984). As O'Hanlon notes, early discussions about the Kuma used the kind of sociological approach that Douglas advocated but introduced a further variable: affinal relations. Mervyn Meggitt (1964) argued that the people whom he studied, the Mae Enga, considered incoming wives as polluting and dangerous because these wives mostly came from enemy groups. In the Kuma case wives were usually from friendly groups and therefore not considered polluting or dangerous. Yet further qualifications are needed here. Meggitt's argument implies a simple determination of cultural notions by features of social structure, but his propositions do not hold when we consider them on a broader front.

First, among the Melpa, or Mt. Hagen, people, who live between the Kuma and the Mae, affinal relations are also generally friendly but there are strong ideas of menstrual pollution (which have continued through many recent social changes). Second, among the Mae themselves, because of the institution of ceremonial exchange between, among others, individual affines, relations at the interindividual level can also be friendly. Third, for the Kuma, at least those studied by O'Hanlon from 1980 onward, it is not true that men are simply unconcerned about female pollution (O'Hanlon 1989, 41 ff.); in fact, North Wall Wahgi Kuma men's ideas on the subject read rather like a mild version of Melpa notions. They do contrast themselves with the Melpa in declaring themselves to be less concerned about menstrual dangers, yet they clearly share important elements of the same worldview as Melpa men have. Both have the idea that sexual intercourse, and especially menstrual contact, can harm male growth patterns and spoil men's skins, which especially should look strong and glossy at dance occasions, rather than ashy and thin (i.e., depleted), as they do after intercourse or polluting contact.

All of these points indicate the relative futility of block contrasts that do not take further features of *both* a social *and* a cultural kind into account. First, the boundaries between types are themselves blurred. Kuma, Melpa, and Enga merge into one another and have done so historically, although the process has presumably speeded up since colonial times. Second, relations that are hostile in some regards or spheres may be friendly in others. And third, the cultural dimension simply cannot be left out of the equations we make. Kuma and Melpa men share many cultural notions, which in turn make their mutual interaction across boundaries easier. Yet the cultural is not the same as the social. The Kuma/Melpa comparison demonstrates this point, showing that friendly affinal relations in social terms do not preclude the existence of ideas of menstrual pollution in cultural terms. Ideas of gender must be attended to in their own right here. Kuma sexual and marriage practices also differ, however, from those of the Melpa and conduce to a lesser overall concern with matters of pollution.

Finally, in this chapter I wish to stress again the significance of history. In Pangia, when I first worked there in 1967, people had recently given up a wide range of menstrual taboos, and individual men often

remarked on their lack of fear of menstrual blood. This apparent abandonment of "traditional" ideas and practices was a result of a campaign
by incoming Lutheran and Catholic missionaries, I was told. My problem thus seemed to be as follows: If such ideas were long established
and traditional, how could they be abolished so easily and swiftly?
Much later, I received a clue to the situation. The major ensemble of
menstrual taboos had been imported into the area around the turn of
the century by ritual experts who were "marketing" a particular circu-
lating cult, the Female Spirit cult, bringing it into Pangia from the Kewa
region to the north. Older men in the 1960s could still remember this
event. The Lutheran missionaries, much later, attacked this cult, and its
abandonment incidentally meant the ending of the prohibitions associated with it. Cultural categories thus themselves have a historical life
span, and ethnotheories of the body are perfectly capable of changing
over time. Interestingly, I find myself here reaching back, beyond Mary
Douglas's work, to that of Mauss, who also argued that concepts of the
person/self (and thus of the body) have changed over time, although
his focus was an evolutionary narrative, while mine is rather on
shorter-scale local histories (*petits récits*, in the words of Lyotard [1984]).

In the next chapter I consider the issues of history, socialization,
change, and memory in greater depth, by comparing the ideas of two
theorists, Pierre Bourdieu and Paul Connerton.

Chapter 2

Habit or Habitus? Theories of Memory, the Body, and Change

Marcel Mauss's work on concepts of the self and the person clearly fed into Mary Douglas's formulations regarding grid and group, as the preceding chapter has indicated. In these formulations the body becomes a repository for social symbolism, a receptacle but also a "natural" model for "mindful" operations. The other strand of Mauss's thinking, on "techniques of the body," gives to the body side of the equation a more active role while stressing that learned forms of bodily action become strongly imprinted and operate at what we may recognize as a subconscious or unconscious level. It is this strand that has been taken up by one of Mauss's successors in the field of comparative sociology, Pierre Bourdieu, and is separately reconsidered also by Paul Connerton in his work on collective aspects of memory. While Connerton's work clearly links with that of Bourdieu, it is perhaps less clear why it is relevant to the study of the body. The answer to this question, however, is to be found in Connerton's interest in "incorporative" acts of remembering, which require the physical involvement of persons, and, at another level, in rethinking what in general we mean by the term *memory*.

Pierre Bourdieu's work shows a consistent concern over time with reformulating materialist-Marxist ideas of society in terms of a theory of socialization or education. He takes up a theme that is also well-known to cognitive psychologists: the different ways in which learning takes place in different societies or cultures (see, e.g., Lancy 1983). In the context of his Kabyle ethnography he is particularly interested in the "look and learn" method of socialization by which practical skills are imparted directly without reaching the level of discourse. Children also watch how adults behave and imitate them (although, of course, they may be subject also to explicit criticism and guidance). Bourdieu's further theoretical argument is that such a form of learning is made easier because of the structural consistency of knowledge patterns. He thus integrates the approach of Lévi-Strauss into his own perspectives through his recognition of these patterns, which Lévi-Strauss saw as structures. But not only is knowledge consistent in a mental sense; among the Kabyle it is also spatially embodied (Bourdieu 1977, 87 ff.), notably in the construction of the Kabyle house. It is this stress on the material and embodied dimension that separates Bourdieu from Lévi-Strauss.

The Kabyle life-world is in this regard somewhat like that of many New Guinea peoples: it is structured by gender and by an honor/shame complex that goes with ideas about gender. The categories of right/left, man/woman, male honor/female honor are all encoded in the spaces of the house. Bourdieu argues that the mental construction of this world of objects does not correspond to a neo-Kantian form of consciousness. Consciousness is turned inside out, and "the mind is a metaphor of the world of objects" (Bourdieu 1977, 89). (The theoretical agenda here is closely tied also to the Durkheimian proposition about the primacy of the social, a line of thinking that also stretches into the work of Jacques Lacan, who argued that the unconscious is itself structured like a language and is in a sense "cultural.") Whether one speaks of "metaphor" here or not, it is clear that Bourdieu is arguing that the representation of mental categories is embodied, in two ways: by the material constructions people make (e.g., houses) and by the positioning of their own human bodies in relation to these constructions. What is achieved overall, he notes, is the integration of body space with cosmic space. Movement outward is seen as male by the Kabyle, movement inward as female. The male sphere is identified with communal religious action, the female with individual magic (rites aimed at domesticating male sexual partners, e.g.). It is apparent that these categories also function as an ideology supporting gender hierarchy.

The function of bodily hexis thus goes beyond simple practical adaptation. The body is in fact treated as a source of encoding memory, and to it is entrusted in mnemonic form fundamental principles of the culture, which are naturalized through being made embodied (a cross-cultural case of "the word made flesh," we might say). Rather than speaking of metaphor at this point, Bourdieu uses the more cogent and concrete idea of metonymy: *pars pro toto,* the body as an index of society. He is careful not to attribute too great a rigidity here. Socialization lays down limits on invention but allows a certain range of variability (Bourdieu 1977, 94). But, through institutionalization of bodily movements and positions, hexis becomes habitus, a master concept for Bourdieu, linking the individual to society. *Habitus* refers both to a general concept in Bourdieu's scheme of thought and to the very specific, local, "emic" ideas of a given people, which he insists we must take into account in order to understand them. He stresses also that cosmic notions always operate in definable practical contexts and are adjusted to the exigencies of practice—for example, in the reckoning of seasons and their relationship to farming work.

Bourdieu expands further his idea of metonymy by referring to *mimesis,* a term that goes back to the ideas of Jane Ellen Harrison on ancient Greek ritual and also prefigures the much more recent writings of Michael Taussig on "mimesis and alterity" (Harrison [1903] 1955; Taussig 1993). As it happens, it is also an idea that finds an antecedent in Mauss's work on magic, in which he writes on bodily movements that accompany magical rituals (see chap. 1). Mimesis is the physical counterpart of metonymy in language, and, as Bourdieu notes, "The most characteristic operations of its logic . . . take the form of movements of the body, turning to the right or left, putting things upside down, going in, coming out, cutting, tying" (1977, 116). Instead of "mentalities" and "hermeneutics," therefore, we are dealing rather with scheme transfers via bodily habitus (as the source of "durable, transposable dispositions," in which we can underline the "transposable" element of the definition). In a brief reference to medical matters Bourdieu notes the applicability of his approach to the study of psychosomatic medicine and its concern with "the language of the organs" (120). He goes on to enunciate a theory of language origins that is shared with many human ethologists, who are interested in the prelinguistic origins of language. Language itself encapsulated bodily meanings and actions, and ritual movements and language show this very clearly.

Bourdieu here touches on a rich vein of ideas that has engrossed philologists, ethologists, and philosophical language theorists (e.g., Johnson 1987). Ritual action relates to the roots of language by reenacting in bodily ways meanings that may otherwise have lost their embodied reference. It also exemplifies exactly the kind of scheme transfer which Bourdieu takes to be central to the workings of the habitus. To take a well-known ethnographic example, when a Trobriand garden magician mimics the action of yams growing in a garden and says, "The belly of my garden swells," he transfers the scheme of pregnancy in the human body over to the scheme of garden fertility, thereby setting up a correspondence that reenergizes both contexts (Malinowski 1935). What is involved here is not just symbolic action based on metaphor but also the bringing together of two separate spheres, which thereby become cosmically fused. The terms *metonymy* and *mimesis* are intended to grasp this process.

Bourdieu sums up his own argument by noting that he has been describing "the socially informed body" with all its "senses" (1977, 124). In those senses the physical and the moral are fused, as in the phrase "sense of duty," and we arrive once more at the mindful body concept of Lock and Scheper-Hughes, adding to it the concept of mimesis as one of the means whereby the mindful body shows itself in the realm of practice.

One criticism that has been made of Bourdieu's early theorizing is that it provides no particular way of explaining social change. The habitus reproduces itself over time unless external events intervene, perhaps. Yet there should also be internal dynamics and contradictions that lead to change. One way in which his scheme can accommodate change is in terms of his idea of "limits on invention." If there are limits, these may be stretched, and, in addition, within them there are variations that may change in emphasis over time. Bloch's study of Malagasy ritual over a long time period exemplifies both this process and the effects of historical events on major emphases in ritual practices (Bloch 1986). In general, also, Bourdieu's approach appears to render moot the question of agency and consciousness. Since he attributes the strongest role in determining action to the habitus, it is unclear what place is left for agency, if by this we mean the conscious ability and propensity to make choices between pathways of action (and thus also at times to pursue and promote change). The same downplaying of agency may go along with, in his treatment, a downplaying of individuality and what Tony Cohen has called "self consciousness" (Cohen 1994). Finally, by the same token questions of morality, as they enter into the choices people make, become hard to handle in Bourdieu's scheme. How are we to understand those numerous cases when people deviate from or actively resist moral injunctions or when they afterward experience remorse?

Paul Connerton's work approaches the problem of change from another perspective, that of commemorative ceremonies, which themselves may alter over time. Like Bourdieu, he sees the body as a vital site of memory on which such ceremonies are based, and at one point he echoes (though, curiously, without citation) Bourdieu's formulation. Bourdieu wrote: "Every group entrusts to bodily automatisms those principles most basic to it and most indispensable to its conservation" (1977, 218). Connerton's version is: "Every group, then, will entrust to bodily automatisms the values and categories which they are most anxious to conserve" (Connerton 1989, 102). (Still more curiously, both formulations were long preceded by that of Thurnwald [see chap. 1]).

One can question the exclusivity of this proposition (are important values always and only entrusted to bodily automatisms?) without doubting its potential applicability to particular cases. Linked to Connerton's formulation is his distinction between three kinds of memory: personal memory belonging to the life histories of individuals, cognitive memory (cultural knowledge), and habit memory, which corresponds to bodily automatisms (1989, 22 ff.). Connerton defines this as "the capacity to reproduce a certain performance" (22) and notes that it has generally been downgraded by philosophers as less truly a mental act or event than memories that people consciously evoke, yet in practical social life it is clearly an important component of "cultural competence." Indeed, in a sense all ordered social interaction depends on it, as do the majority of the practical skills that we use on a routine basis.

From another viewpoint, emphasizing habit and habit memory brings us closer to lived experience than other approaches of a semiotic kind that see cultural meanings inscribed on the body and on clothing that different categories of people wear. Connerton argues that clothing not only conveys messages that can be decoded; it also helps actually to mold character by influencing the body's movements (1989, 33). This is an important observation and one, once more, much in line with Mauss's earlier observations (see chap. 1). Connerton cites here the case of tight corsets worn by European women in the nineteenth century and remarks that the term *straight-laced*, which nowadays simply has a moral reference, derives from this time, when it had a dual bodily and moral significance. This is also in line with Bourdieu's dictum that the command "Stand up straight!" embodies a whole moral code.

Like many theorists of ritual, Connerton is interested in how rituals, while in fact accommodating change, have as their overt purpose the representation of history as unchanging. Commemorative cere-

monies do this by repeatedly referring their participants and spectators
back to primordial events that have become the charter for an ongoing
contemporary state of affairs. In this way rituals deny change, reinvig-
orating the present from the past—in Bourdieu's terms, reproducing
the habitus. Yet they may also prefigure change. Connerton instances
Bakhtin's view of the revolutionary potential of carnival: "For here the
inversions of hierarchic order characteristic of carnival are to be read no
longer as a covert means of reaffirming hierarchy [as in Max Gluck-
man's distinction between *rebellion* and *revolution*], but, on the contrary,
as a mechanism of social liberation in which the device of symbolic representation is employed as leverage" (1989, 50). Carnival is the product
of a kind of social imagination, envisaging a utopia, and this vision can
lead to real change. Connerton recognizes that ritual itself has less
potential for its own internal variance than does myth, and this for a
number of reasons. Liturgical words may depend on invariance for
their perceived power, and this holds a fortiori for the bodily encoding
of performative actions, which he argues form a limited repertoire:
"The body is held braced and attentive in standing; the hands are
folded and placed as though bound in praying; persons bow down and
express their impotence by kneeling. . . . The relative sparseness of such
repertoires is their source of strength," he suggests. This is an interesting claim, which he does not fully elaborate. He does go on to point out
an apparent difference between verbal and nonverbal behavior here.
Thus, to kneel is not just like stating one's subordination. "To kneel in
subordination is to display it through the visible, present substance of
one's body. . . . The elementariness of the repertoire from which such
"sayings" are drawn makes possible at once their performative power
and their effectiveness as mnemonic systems" (57).

Connerton contrasts the subtlety and ambiguity of language here
with the "elementary" codifications that are enacted through the body.
His argument can be both challenged from one viewpoint and supported from another. It can be challenged because language also can
have a performative aspect as an illocutionary act with perlocutionary
effects (Austin 1962). Further, either a linguistic or a nonlinguistic act of
subordination may in fact be a lie, if performed without sincere intent
or it may be contraindicated if the situation later alters. Let us, however, grant the validity of the idea that actions may speak louder than
words in ritual, as in other contexts. Why is this so? Any particular cultural code will have its own specific, and historical, answers to this

question. Most probably, the power of the act will be referred back to the first time it was performed, with the implication that it represents a value firmly rooted, persistent, and therefore "strong," "meaningful." From a theoretical perspective we can also suggest that certain gestures have an ethological component, recapitulating the immediate commu nicative practices of ourselves as a species and of other species also. Animals have repertoires of gestures to communicate dominance, aggression, subordination, playfulness, attraction, care, etc., and, inso- far as our gestures are similarly based, it is from this, perhaps, that they take their power, rather than from their "elementariness." Thus, bow- ing, kneeling, or prostrating oneself clearly is a way of submitting to the other by assuming a posture from which one *cannot* be threatening or combative. It is also a form of appeasement, which we can expect to limit the aggressive response of the dominant other: exactly as one may be enjoined to "crawl" to the boss in hopes of gaining a reprieve after wrongdoing. I would suggest that it is from these ethological sources that the elementary power of bodily symbolism is drawn.

As he acknowledges, Connerton's exposition here draws heavily on that by Rappaport (1979). Rappaport's own insights are, in turn, based partly on those of the linguist Charles S. Peirce and his distinc- tions between varieties of signs as symbols, icons, and indices (Rappa- port 1979, 180). Connerton's citation of the power of indexical action in ritual derives also from Rappaport's creative application of Peirce's ideas to the context of ritual. A kneeling supplicant is an index of his or her own need and in this regard is less likely, perhaps, to be lying whereas, as Rappaport points out, when a sign is linked only arbitrar- ily to what it signifies the possibilities of deception are greatly multi- plied (1979, 180–81).

In this context we are often dealing with both postures and ges- tures. These two forms of action also often form the basis of the identi- fication of the performer in a ritual with the mythical dead whose actions are being recalled, an identification that reaches an appropriate bodily climax in possession, when the ancestors or the heroes take over the bodies of performers who represent them and thus, as Connerton says, represent themselves to the spectators (1989, 69). The actors thus "become" the ancestors, and this could not happen without the union of the ancestral spirits and the *bodies* of the performers. Possession is only an extreme case of the wider phenomenon Connerton identifies here: bodily social memory (71), through which "the past is, as it were, sedimented in the body" (p. 72). Rephrasing the old distinction between literate and nonliterate cultures, he distinguishes between inscribing and incorporating practices. In the former, technical devices retain information, while, in the latter, the human body is the instrument of remembering. The remembering involved is always a reenactment, a restatement of relationships rather than a straightforward cognitive act that can take place in the mind of the individual. Standing up when an important person enters the room provides an example of what Connerton calls "the choreography of authority." It is an act of "remembering" that the person who enters does hold high status; it is also a recognition of this fact in the present and thereby recreates the fact at the moment of action itself. Connerton remarks here on the fact that bodily postures are also incorporated into language, in terms such as *an upright person* or a *person of high standing.*

He distinguishes further between techniques of the body, proprieties of the body, and ceremonies of the body (Connerton 1989, 79). In his usage "techniques" include communicative gestures such as hand movements. While these may exhibit some cross-cultural continuities, there are also differences. One study that compared Italians and Jews in New York found that for the Italians gestures actually constituted a communicative code that could be used without words whereas for the Jews gestures were an accompaniment to, or orchestration of, their words, a mimesis of the words themselves but one not capable of communicating without them (80–81). We might ask here what circumstances conduce to one or the other way of "talking with one's hands." Perhaps the need to exclude others from the process of communication may play a part, since outsiders cannot "read" the hand signals developed by a set of insiders. In general, the category of techniques of the body needs to be expanded to include all learned routines and skills, as Mauss did in his essay (see chap. 1).

Under "proprieties" Connerton lists table manners (discussed also by Lévi-Strauss [1969] and Elias [1978]). Elias shows that, for example, the "proper" uses of knives, forks, and spoons developed in European culture only gradually and that current standards were derived from those followed by the French leisured upper class by the end of the eighteenth century (Connerton 1989, 83). Such rules develop in a context of strong "group" control, in Mary Douglas's sense, and the body again becomes the instrument that links the individual to the context of social control. (I myself remember well the first time I sat as a new Prize

Fellow at the High Table in Trinity College Cambridge in 1965, and was slightly baffled by an array of forks beside my plate. I must have picked up one that was not right for the moment, and the very senior fellow at my side, Kitson Clark, rebuked me. His implication was that I was not properly socialized for such an "upper class" setting. The anecdote underlines the point that "manners" of this sort are defined from the top downward and represent a class-based cultural hegemony, an aspect that is explored in detail by Bourdieu in his discussion of "taste" [Bourdieu 1984]). One can also comment here that proprieties are from another point of view also techniques, since they must be learned, and that such appropriate techniques further enter as elements into the category of ceremonies. Eating at the "High Table" is thus an exercise in the use of techniques to demonstrate proprieties that form part of a representational ceremony emphasizing the difference between Fellows of the College and their students, a difference picked out also by the type of gowns worn by Fellows and by the kinds of food and wine served to them.

This ceremony of eating together at the High Table was one of the few mechanisms whereby social position and manners were impressed on the members of the College as a whole, including its new Fellows. Since induction into the position of Fellow was by intellectual merit (especially, perhaps, in the newly meritocratic days of the 1960s) persons of different backgrounds—though still all male at that time—were regularly brought into this sphere of College life and thus carried with them the danger of disrupting the existing "habitus." Such is the hegemonic significance of "class" in English social life that an emphasis on matters such as table manners could actually function as a mechanism of control, precisely as Connerton in his more experience-distant way notes for the rules of eighteenth-century court society. It is in this kind of context, also, that a habit becomes a rule, since it must be taught anew to incoming members of the group who may not have acquired it as a part of their earlier class-based socialization. For the sake of the privileges involved—not least the quality of the food—most initiates, like myself, are only too willing to fall in with the rules (habits) as they stand, and it is this kind of bodily resocialization that Connerton is referring to in his general argument at the end of the introduction to his book, in which he states that "there is an inertia in social structures that is not adequately explained by any of the current orthodoxies of what a social structure is" (5; cf. 102). My own example here indicates another point: *inertia* is perhaps too passive a term for a process that is actively reproduced by those in control on occasions that otherwise might not seem to have anything to do with their authority. Such occasions are contexts in which Mary Douglas's insight applies well: the social body does constrain the perception of the physical body.

A feature that is interesting in such contexts of control is the continuous cross-over, in fact, between the physical and the social. Connerton's example here is that of blood, a concept that in the European case is linked to hierarchy, in the same way as is the theme of table manners. A lineage name, a personal name, a coat of arms, all "allude in a somewhat etherealised manner to something that is distinctly and directly corporeal: blood" (Connerton 1989, 86). Blood comes to be a symbol in this way because it stands for the reproduction of estates. It is a "preclass" symbol that is transmuted into taste or distinction once a class-society comes into being. Its European use in an aristocratic social structure is paralleled in principle by its widespread use in more egalitarian social structures as a means of differentiating either groups or networks of kinsfolk. Among the Melpa of Papua New Guinea blood is one among a set of substance-based concepts that define both unity and difference between people. *Mema tenda wamb* are primarily those who have a kinship link mediated by females, since female blood is held to be wrapped by semen in the womb at conception, but the term can *also* refer at times to the solidarity of all those who belong to a single group (A. J. Strathern 1972). In this shift we see an example of the crossover from the body to the social group. The social group is represented as in fact being a single body in respect to a shared element, blood, and certain kinship rules and practices are thereby implied. Fundamental rules of filiation, inheritance, marriage, and so on are encoded in this way, just as the link between "rank" and "blood" encoded the idea of patrimonial estates in Europe. "To the manner/manor born" is the phrase that in turn encapsulates this point and reflects also the fact that bodily hexis communicates social class, sometimes at an unconscious level, even if clothing or wealth does not.

Connerton returns here to his focus on habit memory. Such memory is expressed in smooth performances, and these may be the product of many awkward ones. It is this sense of habit as the product of prior learning that Connerton wishes to highlight, and perhaps that is why he chooses his term *habit* rather than simply echoing Bourdieu's revivified term *habitus*. At this point in his text he gives a number of references both to Foucault and to Bourdieu in the textual notes, yet he does not appropriate Bourdieu's terminology. Bourdieu's discursive use of the term *habitus* makes it rather difficult to pin down a difference between his work and Connerton's in this regard. For Bourdieu habitus is, for example, "the durably installed generative principle of regulated improvisations," or "history turned into nature," or the "immanent law, *lex insita*, laid down in each agent by his earliest upbringing," or a set of "durable, transposable dispositions" (Bourdieu 1977, 78 ff.). The overall emphasis appears to be on the fact of early socialization and on the unconscious character of the disposition that is produced, a character that conduces to the maintenance and transmission of the form of conduct in question.

Connerton's specifications for *habit* can be compared here. "Habits are more than technical abilities," he writes (Connerton 1989, 93), because they are the products of inclination and desire and are thus affective. "A habit is more than a disposition" he adds. A disposition may indicate a latent tendency to act in a certain way, but a habit is the act itself, as it is repeated over time. Connerton here uses "habit" in a way that sits halfway between Bourdieu's theoretical construction, the habitus, and Bourdieu's own concept of "practice." Finally, and most important for Connerton, "habit is not just a sign" (94). In this regard, and following Bourdieu, he is objecting to both structuralism and the linguistic model of society that informs it (a model that has influenced many, including the psychiatrist Jacques Lacan). As with the preeminence accorded "cognitive memory," as against "habit memory," this stress on actions as signs is taken by Connerton as a kind of imperialistic "mentalism." Opposition to such a mentalism is thus mounted in terms of a concentration on the body, and habit memory is located in the body. Connerton also argues consistently that formality and performativity, expressed in bodily hexis, are highly significant for the understanding of ritual and that therefore embodiment rather than "text" is the key to analyses of ritual. It is the "etherealization" of the body to which he objects. At the end of his book he makes the point most clearly, and in a way that associates him with Bourdieu and with the phenomenological influences on Bourdieu's thought and differentiates them both from the work of Mary Douglas. The body is socially constituted not just in the sense that "it is constructed as an object of knowledge or discourse," but also because "it is culturally shaped in its actual practices and behaviour" (104)—exactly as Mauss noted long ago.

In seeking a difference between Connerton's and Bourdieu's work we can say, then, that it rests on a rather fine distinction between *habit* and *habitus.* Using a turn of expression from Bourdieu himself, we could say that habit is the *opus operatum,* while habitus is its modus operandi; or we could note that "habit" is a descriptive category to which Connerton gives analytical content, while "habitus" in Bourdieu's writings attains the status of a theoretical construct, a hidden key to understanding. Neither concept, however, solves for us questions of change, since in both it is reproduction, continuity, or inertia that is stressed. Yet, in choosing his examples from European, and especially French, history, Connerton is certainly also implying that habits change over time and that social meanings are continuously re-encoded in differing forms of bodily hexis. In practice, at all stages of one's life certain new forms of hexis are adopted, a point that indicates the plasticity of people and makes it possible to accommodate the idea of change. Our bodies and minds are clearly very complex layerings of different times and kinds of learning and habit formation, and certain types of habit may be harder to discard than others, so that at any time we literally encode our own histories. But, if this is so, it also underlines the fact that we do indeed inhabit "mindful bodies" and that Bourdieu and Connerton are right to reject the (implicitly Cartesian) mentalism that informs the semiotic or linguistic theory of society.

In the course of their discussions of bodily skills Bourdieu (1977, 20) and Connerton (1989, 95) both refer to the work of the phenomenologist Maurice Merleau-Ponty. Merleau-Ponty in fact provides a philosophical basis for the views of the body that both Bourdieu and Connerton implicitly construct. Bourdieu takes such a viewpoint for granted with his idea of habitus, while Connerton more clearly situates it in his concrete notion of habit. The viewpoint is that the body, in Mauss's terms, is an apt "instrument" for the social operations that are performed on it and by means of it. Merleau-Ponty's aim is broader. It is to show that all of our mental operations in fact are constrained by the characteristics of our bodies. He is therefore concerned to break away from the Cartesian basis of phenomenology that was at first espoused by Husserl and also to break out of the realm of words (as does Connerton) and get back to bodily experience. Merleau-Ponty's work is thus important for us here, although his purpose is different from my own. Whereas I am largely concerned with cross-cultural comparisons and use as my data categories that are already "constructed," Merleau-Ponty wants to lay down a general basis for the study of perception that will transcend cultural categories as such.

Yet his work certainly incorporates culture in its foundations, since he argues that perception always depends on a field or context that enhances or reduces ambiguity and, hence, that perception cannot be reduced to pure sense impressions (Langer 1989, 5). Such a "field" already incorporates cultural factors, and the implication is that, if these factors vary, so will perception. Equally, memory is involved and hence prior learning, the "horizon of the past." Perception involves selection and thus also both a focus of attention on certain features and a judgment about those features; in other words it is inherently subjective in a certain sense, or, rather, it is "intersubjective" (18).

Merleau-Ponty's most valuable contribution was to show the influence of spatiotemporal factors on perception, through the concepts of perspective, field, and horizon. Here his efforts perhaps dovetail with the propositions of quantum mechanics and with general relativity. In any case his aim is to remove the concept of the body as an object and the mechanistic physiology that goes with such a concept and to reintroduce the body as our "point of view upon the world" (Langer 1989, 25). He wants also to go beyond the psychophysical position that we make psychic representations about objective events that occur in our "real bodies." Merleau-Ponty points out that medical patients who have lost a limb can still sometimes feel it and that this means that their perceptions are conditioned by their personal, bodily memories (a type of habit memory, in Connerton's terms). But this also implies that we must see the totality of the person as the locus for such memories and cannot adhere to a sharp distinction between the psychic and the physical, as Descartes did. The phantom limb phenomenon was in fact recognized by Descartes himself, and he saw too that the hypothetical "union of soul and body," which was his unsolved problem, is one that is readily perceived by the senses (Langer 1989, 30). The phenomenon underlines the historically layered character of the body and therefore of perception itself, and Merleau-Ponty distinguishes between the "habitual body" and the "present body" in recognition of this point. As Langer notes in her commentary and exegesis of Merleau-Ponty's work, "We all carry our past with us insofar as its structures have become "sedimented" in our habitual body" (33). The formulation here exactly fits those of both Bourdieu and Connerton. Bourdieu's work is even more foreshadowed in another statement by Langer about "recognizing the dialectical movement of our existence," a movement that carries biological existence into the personal and "allows the personal and the cultural to become sedimented in general, anonymous structures" (34). Insofar as Langer is glossing Merleau-Ponty here, it is clear that we have identified him as a philosophical precursor of Bourdieu, a common sense proposition given Bourdieu's extensive knowledge of the history of phenomenological thought from Hegel onward.

Merleau-Ponty's concept of the body image also foreshadows the mindful body theme. Body image is not just a set of impressions about an objective body. Rather, it incorporates the "project" of the subject and therefore is an image of "incarnate intentionality" (Langer 1989, 40), operating with "the world" as its horizon. Hence the notion of "being-in-the-world" (similar to Heidegger's idea of Dasein). Perception has to do with figure-background formations, which are always conditioned by the position of the observer's body, and this fact can therefore never be omitted—as also by full functioning of the brain. Such an argument is well fitted to the analysis of habits, and Merleau-Ponty argues that acquiring these is like fitting objects and the body together. He uses a good example: adjustment to an unfamiliar car. Apart from the details of this process, it has a gestalt quality, which has exactly the sense of incorporating the car into one's body, and this process is necessary for good judgment in practical driving. If one has to use two differently structured cars in the course of a single day, one soon discovers this point. Here one experiences not phantom limbs but phantom clutches and gear sticks or reaches to switch on the lights only to find that the switch is somewhere else. Generalizing from such an example leads to the point that the body "is essentially an expressive space" through which other expressive spaces come into existence, and so "bodily spatiality . . . is the very condition for the coming into being of a meaningful world" (Langer 1989, 47).

Finally, here we may note that for Merleau-Ponty there is no realm of pure reflection such as Descartes envisaged, hence there is no pure cogito to use as the foundation of knowledge. The phenomenological cogito that he proposes instead is one that emphatically locates us in the intersubjective and temporal world. In this regard not only does the body become mindful, as we have already seen, but the mind becomes fully embodied. "Prior to any philosophizing, there is that comprehensive, pre-personal experience in which the body-subject comes into being by simultaneously grasping the world and itself" (Langer 1989,

121). This is the prereflective cogito that Merleau-Ponty has been at pains to establish through his inquiry into the nature of perception. We can use it as a general, cross-cultural category while recognizing that the concept already implies variation, since each world that is grasped is a culturally different one. It is in any case a statement of the union of soul and body that Descartes sought vainly to explicate, and it achieves its solution to Descartes's problem by abolishing it in favor of a primordial totality. It is worth noting also that Merleau-Ponty's scheme allows in a sense for a more creative role of the body than does Bourdieu, since he grants to it a creative, gestural, intentionality that contributes to the overall agency of the human person.

Chapter 3

Mind, Body, and Soul

As I have remarked in the introduction, contemporary efforts to reconceptualize the person or the self around or against the mind-body dichotomy have conventionally associated the figure of Descartes with the inception of this dichotomy. Several questions arise here: first, what was the cultural and intellectual background against which Descartes was himself working? Second, what was his own intentional reworking of that background? Third, was his influence at first confined to the educated literati, and, if so, how did it then come to have the encompassing influence that it is usually credited with? Finally, how would matters look if, instead of regarding Descartes's work within the traditions of European philosophy, we were to make the basic anthropological analytical move and compare his ideas relativistically with those developed in other cultural traditions over time?

The last question here is the one that I think is in fact potentially the most illuminating, because it avoids essentializing the discussion in terms of a single pursuit of putatively universal truth. The earlier questions can also aid in the process of relativizing Descartes's ideas, since elucidation of them can show in what ways his work represented a twist on existing modes of thought, developed within European Christendom. I cannot, however, deal with all these questions in detail here.

The overall point is that Descartes utilized an existing religious dichotomy and turned it into a philosophical one, thus at the same time justifying a religious notion by means of philosophy and, more covertly, bolstering philosophy through an appeal to essentially religious notions: a kind of double twist, giving his writings a Janus-faced aspect, but enabling him to draw on tradition while significantly transforming it. Basically, his act was to conflate "soul" with "mind." (As David Parkin has, with characteristic acuity, pointed out, Descartes's treatment of this matter was actually rather ambiguous and complex,

since at times he sees mind and soul as the same and at times as different, depending on his purposes [1985, 136–38.]).

Relativizing or contextualizing Descartes's work in this way can
help us to explore both its specificity and its historical impact. First,
Descartes was operating within a framework of Christian theology that
required that both God and humanity remain central in the cosmos.
Second, within the Christian tradition he had to address himself to the
problem that, if God made man in his own (male?) likeness, then God
also must have a body, and how could his essence be kept pure from
bodily corruption? Various answers are possible (e.g. distinguishing
between a pure, pre-Fall and an impure, post-Fall body), but
Descartes's answer concentrated on the soul-body opposition. Making
the soul absolutely distinct from the body, and relating the soul to God
(as in Neoplatonism) was a means of ensuring a region of purity for
both God and man. But in that case the solution preferred now fell victim to the questions addressed to Descartes by Princess Elizabeth of
Bohemia—namely, if soul and body are so different, how can the soul
move the body? And also, how can thoughts be so susceptible to influence from the emotional or bodily state of the person? Descartes's
answer, that there is a union of soul and body in which both thought
and imagination intermingle, turned his own dyad back into a kind of
triad, raising questions in turn about the kind of totality so constructed
as the third realm of experience. In fact, this third realm is much closer
to the single realm later argued for by the phenomenologist Merleau-
Ponty, as we have seen (chap. 2) but Merleau-Ponty does not base this
realm on any preexisting dichotomy. Descartes's ad hoc solution to his
problem is thus in a sense taken as an ontological starting point by Merleau-Ponty, not as a philosophical coda to a major dichotomy set up in
a priori terms.

The translation of Descartes's writings on the soul and the body
into a secularized mind-body problem, in which the theological content
of the idea of the soul is expunged, must have taken place at least in
part through the work of Immanuel Kant in his *Critique of Pure Reason*
(1781). Kant further intellectualized Descartes's ideas and provided a
framework of logical categories of mind in terms of which the world
was supposedly apprehended, thus bringing together science and philosophy and paving the way for nineteenth-century physics. It is puzzling, therefore, why we do not speak of Kantianism as much as of
Cartesianism. The answer again probably lies in the historical fact of a

specific school of writers arising who identified themselves as Cartesians and further sharpened the original soul-body dichotomy as a secular philosophical position stripped of its theological underpinnings.

For the anthropologist these historical points underline again the advantage of a relativizing strategy. From this viewpoint it is not so much a matter of who is right that is at issue but of how to compare systems of thought. The Melpa people of Papua New Guinea, for example, sought to explain the mind-body problem in a way analogous to Descartes's solution via the pineal gland. They see the mind-body interaction as taking place in the *noman*. But the Melpa *noman* is not like Descartes's "soul." For one thing it is separate from the soul, or life force (*min*); for another it is the (or *a*) seat of emotions as well as of thought. And, finally, the connections between the *noman* and the rest of the person are intimate and direct, since serious sickness begins in the *noman*. From this example we can see also what is gained and lost by different cross-cultural conceptualizations. The Melpa "project" is the reverse of Descartes's: how to link rather than separate mind and body. That makes their dualistic concepts closer in operation to the holistic ideas of the phenomenologists.

I will return at greater length to the Melpa and other New Guinea peoples later. In this chapter, however, I trace the development of some ideas regarding the soul/body/mind triad in European traditions, particularly in the Greek and Roman traditions as these became enmeshed with Christian ideas over time. This will both enable us partly to situate Descartes's project historically and to indicate the pitfalls involved in translating concepts from one language to another as we look at the changing conflations and distinctions between categories.

The title of Richard Onians's massive work on early European thought conveys the scope of his topic: "The origins of European thought about the body, the mind, the soul, the world, time, and fate" (1954). We can note here the triadic division between body, soul, and mind and their linkage to cosmic matters such as time and fate. The most striking impression one gains from his vigorous exposition is the anchoring of ideas about the person in the body itself such that he depicts a body that is "mindful" in all the senses used by Lock and Scheper-Hughes. Onians' main focus is on early (i.e., for him "Homeric" Greek) society, prior to the efflorescence of democracy and philosophy in fifth century B.C. Athens.

He begins with consciousness and shows how this was linked with various organs and functions of the body. Consciousness was associated with speaking and speaking equated with thinking, being located in the *phrēn* or *phrenes* (pl.) which Onians convincingly argues originally refers not to the diaphragm but to the lungs. Onians at once shows his comparative interests by comparing the Homeric view of thought as speech with the Trobriand concept of *nanola*, intelligence that resides in the larynx and is linked to the ability to learn magical formulae (1954, 14). He identifies also another feature that is commonly found in the concepts of Pacific peoples: an association between thinking and feeling that stresses their processual interdependence rather than their logical separation (we may recall at once that "separation" was the solution Descartes opted for). He suggests that over time the concept of knowing became more detached from its emotional linkages, and the realm of intellect and pure cognition became established (18). Here he shows an evolutionism in his thinking that I will reject but that clearly also belongs to the Cartesian schema. We can see, therefore, how Onians, intent on reaching back to early Greek concepts, in a sense unconsciously passes through the Cartesian moment and carries it into his data. He does not seem to notice that he is comparing "Homeric" culture at large, at least as reflected in the poetry of Homer himself, with the specialized works of philosophers such as Plato and Aristotle. He also exhibits that curious self identification with the classical Greeks that so affected scholars in the nineteenth and first half of the twentieth century, claiming that "we" are more restrained than the early Greeks or *"les primitifs"* (he has just quoted from Lévy-Bruhl, who publicized the notion of the prelogical mentality of primitive people). Yet he recognizes that the so-called primitives may have had the greater phenomenological insight (bringing them into alignment again with Merleau-Ponty), since "there is perhaps no such thing as "un phénomène intellectual ou cognitif pur" for us either. . . . [Yet] . . . we lack terms like *phronein* for the complex unity *that is the reality"* (20; my emph.). *Phronein* is a verb that denotes acts of thinking and feeling, cognition and conation, seen as a single process.

Thinking and emotions were said to be felt in the *phrenes* but also in the heart *(kēr)* or "blood vapor" *(thūmos)*. *Phrenes* Onians interprets as the lungs, the seat of breath, and thus plausibly tied to speech (hence to thinking) (Onians 1954, 27). We see the impact of humoral categories here, since conditions of dryness or wetness were regarded as important for both the *phrenes* and the *thūmos* within them. Sleep was conceived of as a mist coming to the *phrenes*, described as *meliphrōn*, "honey to the *phrenes*." In their efficient, active state, by contrast, the *phrenes* were "dry." In grief or yearning it was thought that "the relevant parts of the body 'melt' and as they diminish there issues liquid" (33), as for example tears. Love also could be conceived of as finding its way into the lungs and melting them. Strong emotions are therefore seen as "wet," while more balanced or ratiocinative states are seen as dry (37).

Since the *thūmos* was considered to be in the *phrenes*, it is reasonable to consider that it is to be translated as "breath" (Onians 1954, 44), or, more precisely, blood vapor, the mist that arises from hot blood. If persons "eat" their own *thūmos*, they will consume their source of strength, rather than renewing it by consuming food and wine. Onians completes another circle here by pointing out that, if the "stuff of consciousness" is breath that arises from blood, we can understand the linkage made between "blood" and "character" (a motif that has many obvious ramifications in European history but here seems to find its origin in a particular ethnotheory of the body). *Thūmos* clearly also carries a sense of willpower (spirit, in this sense), and so energy (*menos*) and courage (*tharsos*) were held to depend on *thūmos*. Courage and anger are both breathed out. (Onians jumps here to Latin, to remind us that "inspiration" is to be seen as drawn from the same basic schema.) There is little doubt that there is a phenomenological basis for all of these expressions, since emotional states are often accompanied by different breathing patterns. Onians himself quotes both William James and Carl Jung in support of the phenomenological reality expressed in these Greek ideas (53). Resonances also occur with New Guinea concepts: the Wiru people of Pangia, for example, consider that anger resides primarily in the nose and can be blown out, thus preventing serious conflict between people. The term for anger in Pangia, in fact, is *nose* (*timini*). (Compare the expression "breathing fire and slaughter.") Finally, the libations of blood that were given to dead souls, to enable them to speak, could work only for those souls who still possessed *phrenes*, or lungs. This part of the ethnotheory of the body explains, therefore, also the use of blood libations in sacrifice.

Other internal organs of the body were also considered the seats of specific capacities. Anger, *cholos*, was literally seen as bile, which could enter the heart and lungs but emerged from the liver. The liver itself was the organ struck by the most painful emotions and hence "came to be regarded as the inmost spring of the deeper emotions." Thoughts and cares, seen as arrows shot by the gods, could pierce the liver and were imaged as *kēres*, small winged creatures. Breath was thought to enter the liver and replenish it, via the *thūmos*, and so help to heal it. The liver thus seems to have been given a passive agency while the stomach, *gastēr*, was credited with active appetite, for food, drink, and also sexual activity. In love, therefore, desire was felt in the stomach but longing and pain in the liver (Onians 1954, 85). Overall here we see not just the attribution of feeling to specific organs but a picture of how these organs interacted in producing emotional syndromes in the person and also how they could be affected by outside agencies such as the gods, via the action of *kēres*. The meaning given to the liver as a seat of deep and often painful emotions, signaled by its production of bile, is also interesting because the liver is an organ of importance in divinatory practices in a number of cultures (see, e.g., Hoskins 1993) and in some instances is reserved for consumption by males (e.g., among the Duna of Papua New Guinea).

We have looked at the interplay of thought and feeling through their concrete location in organs of the body but not at any part of the person that was held to survive death. This shows us very clearly that for the Homeric and post-Homeric Greeks the mind is certainly not to be equated with the soul. The element identifiable with soul was *psuchē* and, as Onians remarks, this is usually linked with breath (as, differently, was *thūmos*), since the verb *psuchoō* means "I blow" (Onians 1954, 93). Despite this dual association with breath, Onians insists that *thūmos* and *psuchē* were not equated. Although *psuchē* was seen as present in the living person, it became active only in death, flying out of the body via the mouth and traveling to Hades, where it became an *eidōlon*, the simulacrum of the once living person (94), similar to visions that appeared in dreams. The precise association, then, may not be with breath as actively energized in life but, rather, with a gaseous or vaporous entity that could be blown out of the body at the point of death. Such a vapor could be analogous to darkness, which was also thought to be a substancelike vapor and not just an absence of light. We see here the importance of a minute reading of texts to extract the exact distinctions that were made, an exercise equally called for in interpretations of ethnographically reported ideas from elsewhere in the world and also of terms in European languages such as *âme, esprit, Seele,* and *Geist,* whose meanings are often seen against the background of Greek and Roman terms. In addition, it must be remembered here that these latter terms were subject to continuous revision over the centuries. Here, following Onians, we have been trying to reconstruct their earlier referents, as shown in the Homeric poems and also in the work of the tragic dramatists such as Aeschylus some centuries after Homer.

Onians adds another point. *Psuchē* was "associated more particularly with the head." The head, in fact, was seen as sacred, and Onians suggests that this means it was felt to be the seat of life itself. If so, however, it must be in a different way from the complex of *phrenes* and *thūmos* in the central part of the body. The quotations Onians gives suggest equally that *head* means the whole person with his or her dignity, status, and decision-making power. It would thus be used in a synecdochal sense. When Zeus nodded his head, the heavens shook. Onians himself notes that "the head is in some sense the person" (1954, 98). If so, it is surely the person seen as a talking, decision-making entity— hence, perhaps, the use of the skull in divinatory consultations with the dead, such as were directed to the prophetic head of the hero Orpheus after his body had been torn to pieces (102). *Psuchai* (pl.) of the dead are represented as standing at the heads of dreamers also. Sneezes, proceeding suddenly from the head, could be taken as prophetic, since they were a sign of disturbance in the *psuchē* within the head. By synecdoche, again, the hair could be taken as a seat of the soul or as a substitute for it, and death was sometimes represented in poetry as the action of the death god in cutting a lock of hair (108).

The final point here is that the head was seen as the seat of life in another, concrete sense as the vessel of the procreative seed or semen, transmitted to the male testes via the cerebrospinal column. The generative seed or fluid was also thought to be carried in the knees, hence the practice of clasping the knees in supplication for mercy (Onians 1954, 174). The association of head with semen also explains the form of representations of the god Hermes as a phallus with a head at the top. Hermes was generative power, also the "giver of increase, wealth" (122). It was thus appropriate that he was the guide of souls *(psuchopompos)* on their journey to Hades.

Onians then traces transitions from these earlier ideas to later ones in which the *psuchē* began to take on functions at first accorded the *phrenes* and *thūmos*, a shift from one part of the body to another. This upward shift in ethnolocation was the prerequisite for the possibility of conflating soul with mind in relation to the brain. Greek ideas thus seem to have moved from a dynamic complexity to a more consolidated, hierarchical picture, aided by the original synecdoche of the head as person and by the particular idea that the head is holy because it is the seat of vital seed. What is left quite unexplained in this treatment is how the heads of women were conceptualized.

It is a part of Onians's overall argument that many aspects of Greek, and also Roman, concepts can be found also in Celtic and Germanic traditions and thus form a generalized backdrop to the development of European thought. It is therefore quite logical for him to switch from the *psuchē* to the Latin terms *anima* and *animus* (which, I have noted, underly the French term *âme* used by Descartes). Roman culture was influenced by Greek textual traditions, a fact that complicates discussions. Onians, however, argues that for the Romans, independently of the Greeks, the "vital principle" was originally thought of as in the head and was described as the "genius" and also the anima. Animus, by contrast, was not the principle of life "but the principle of consciousness" (Onians 1954, 168). This distinction parallels that between *psuchē* and *thūmos. Anima,* he argues, is a generic term like *wind,* while *animus* referred to consciousness within the *praecordia,* or lungs (170). *Animus* is thus also linked with *spiritus,* or breath, in the located sense and connected with intentionality (as seen in the verb *conspiro,* "I conspire," literally "breathe together"). Catching the last breath of a dying person (*postremum spiritum ore excipere*) was therefore an act of taking the mind stuff of the person, which would otherwise be lost. It was not the anima that was caught, since this was blown out and became the immortal part of the person. Onians, in one of his sudden comparative shifts, points out that the idea involved here is paralleled from the Society Islands (Tahiti), where a successor was expected to place his mouth over the mouth of his dying predecessor and thereby gain his knowledge (a dogma that would suit well a chiefly society, we may add).

Onians thus manages to disentangle animus from anima, and it is interesting to note that this means a distinction between mind and soul that exactly parallels not only the early Greek concepts but also, fortuitously, those of the Melpa of Papua New Guinea in their contrast between *noman* and *min.* It is also clear, however, that the similarity of the terms *animus* and *anima* could easily conduce to their conflation and, indeed, may reflect some tendency to such conflation from the outset. We need not suppose that cultural notions were always clear-cut at any stage of their history. Insofar as the Latin terms found their way eventually into the concepts of medieval Christendom, it is clear that their co-identification could again conduce toward the equation in one way or another of soul with mind later made by Descartes.

Before considering the history of Christian ideas, however, I want to take note of the ideas of two other thinkers, one earlier and one later than Onians: Jane Ellen Harrison and Ruth Padel. Jane Harrison was a contemporary of Greek scholars such as Gilbert Murray and Arthur Verrall who began to apply anthropological insights into the history of Greek tragic and comic drama. Her life span, 1850–1928, also over-lapped with that of Émile Durkheim, and she was tremendously influenced by Durkheim's theory of collective representations and religion as a projection of group consciousness, a theory that seems to have been out of favor with some of her English contemporaries. This basic concern of Harrison's shows throughout her whole work and influenced her attitude toward questions about the soul. Her combination of Durkheimian and Frazerian concepts led her to see all ancient art in Greece as concerned originally with the drama of seasonal ritual, the death and rebirth of the *eniautos-daimōn*, the year god. Such a *daimōn* was essentially a projection of the group itself and, therefore, in the primordial sense was its soul. In locating her ideas in this fashion, Harrison ruled out for herself the detailed, persistent pursuit of ethnotheories of the body such as are found in Onians's work. She also used a great deal of evidence not from texts, as Onians tends to do, but from visual art, vases, funeral scenes, and such, perhaps thus tapping into layers of culture lying outside of textual materials and closer to popular conceptions. Since the evidence is not textual, she has perforce to use her own imagination to interpret it and, in doing so, calls on anthropological theory (Harrison [1903] 1955, [1912, 1921] 1962). She does make references to the question of the individual soul, as, for example, when she writes on a scene depicting mourning executed on a vase of the archaic period (prior to the fifth century B.C.):

> Within the grave-mound the vase-painter has drawn what he believes to be there, two things—in the upper part of the mound a crowd of little fluttering Keres, and below the single figure of a snake. The Keres are figured as what the Greeks called *eidōla*, little images, shrunken men, only winged. They represent the shadow-soul, strengthless and vain; but the *thūmos* of the man, his strength, his *menos*, his *mana*, has passed into the *daimon* of life and reincarnation, the snake. An *eidolon*, an image, informed by *thūmos*, makes

up something approximately not unlike that complex, psychological conception, our modern immortal soul. (Harrison [1921] 1962,
291, correcting her earlier [1903] 1955, 235)

We can see from this passage ways in which Harrison's formulation *diverges* from that later made by Onians. She thinks of the *thūmos* as
entering the *eidolōn*, whereas Onians urges that it did not, being mortal
consciousness, not the source of life itself, the *psuchē*. *Kēres*, in Onians's
usage, were also attacking spirits, sent by deities, rather than shrunken
eidōla of the dead. Harrison is here attempting two things: to interpret a
grave scene and to link her interpretation to the supposed "modern"
conception of the soul. Onians, by contrast, is intent to uncover the earliest forms of the ethnotheory of the person-body complex. But Harrison also brings in another element: her theory that the individual soul,
however constituted, at death joined the group *daimōn*, in this instance
a snake, which often figured as the incarnation of a deity, such as Zeus
Meilichios (Harrison [1903] 1955, 18). The individual soul is thus made
a part of the deity, who is like a group soul. Harrison thus presents her
data in the context of her picture of the Greek cosmos as a whole.
    This kind of concern is shared also by Ruth Padel. Padel further
takes issue with the evolutionism that underlies the prose of both Onians and Harrison (children of their times, as we all are). The time span
on which she concentrates is the fifth century B.C. (the point at which
Onians by and large leaves off). Her basic image is of the body boundary and of defenses against incursions into it from the outside realm of
"divinity" (generally signaled by the term *daimōn*, which is also important for Harrison). Her inquiry also has as its aim the elucidation of
Greek tragic drama—hence, much of her evidence comes from the
plays of Aeschylus, Sophocles, and Euripides—but her discussion
broadens into a general consideration of the Greek cosmos. The god
Hermes is significant to her theme as the marker of thresholds and also
the one who guides people across thresholds as well as the interpreter
of signs and meanings (hence "hermeneutics" [see also Crapanzano
1992]. As Padel writes: "All this suggests that in Greek culture the contrast between inside and outside for which Hermes stands interprets
other contrasts. . . . Male and female, outside and inside, culture and
nature: these pairings today provide obvious ways of approaching
another thought-world" (1992, 9). Her approach thus combines Oni-

ans's attention to ethnographic minutiae with a perspective derived from structuralist and feminist writings.

For example, she reconsiders the significance of the inner organs of the body in relation to the emotions, noting the term *splanchna*, or "innards," which encompasses the heart, liver, lungs, gallbladder, and vessels (Padel 1992, 13). *Splanchna* in general are the seat of emotions and of overall character. While Onians commits himself strongly to the idea that early Greek ideas were physical and not "metaphorical," Padel is less insistent on the point for fifth-century Athenians. But most of the references do have a physical ring about them. *Splanchna* have feelings, but also hide them, hence their use in divinatory sacrifices in which they were unfolded by a seer in order to be "read" (15). The seer "divided" the entrails in order to "discern" hidden truths impressed on them by outside divinities, who also induced thoughts and feelings in the innards of humans. Hence, consciousness and thinking for the Greeks had their material seats in these same innards, and the tragic poets show their continuity with Homer in this regard (18).

The heart (*kēr, etor,* or *kardia*) was seen as mobile and shaken by emotions, while the liver (*hēpar*) was a center of divinatory attention, as a seat especially of anger and fear, and was torn or gashed, for example, by desire. Her account here follows that of Onians. On the much-disputed term *phrenes* she notes the polemic of a Greek doctor who wished to attribute consciousness to the brain rather than to the heart and the *phrenes*. But in popular thought the *phrenes* were still held to be the passive containers of "emotion, practical ideas and knowledge" (Padel 1992, 21). They could also be seen as an active force guiding the *thūmos*, or spirit, always with both an emotional and an intellectual dimension. Loss of *phrenes* meant madness. They were washed also with liquids, such as blood and bile, or gall (*cholos* or *cholē*, black bile, equated with anger). Again, Padel eschews an exclusively physicalist interpretation of words as well as the evolutionist argument that concrete precedes abstract. She cites the semantic space occupied by the Ilongot concept of *liget*, "anger," as comparable to the meanings of the Greek terms she discusses (25) (see Rosaldo 1980). With these precautions she embarks on *thūmos, psuchē,* and *nous* (spirit, soul, and mind).

Thūmos, she notes, derives from *thuo,* "I seethe or boil." It connotes the active, the conative, aspect of the person and can sometimes also be translated as "courage" (Padel 1992, 27) as well as "anger." It collects in and fills the *phrenes*. Its range of reference is complex, and Padel decides that no single translation term will cover it, though she recognizes that the component of breath in its meaning is important, comparing the Latin *spiritus*. One point is clear: the *thūmos* is always located precisely within the body and it moves or is moved within that space. On the whole the presentation is consistent with Onians's argument that *thumos* was originally blood vapor, but Padel's approach to semantics is more subtle than Onians's.

Psuchē also presents a puzzle, she says. While in Onians's account *psuchē* and *thūmos* are differentiated, in Padel's they tend to overlap. This in itself may reflect a process by which *psuchē* took into itself elements formerly attached to *thūmos*. In Plato's usage this process finds its culmination, since the *psuchē* becomes identified with the self and the question of its immortality becomes existentially tantalizing. In other sources it can be "appetitive, perceptive, mobile, intelligent, 'life,' 'self,' 'mind,' 'soul,' ghost," and here she adds a fundamental problem of translation, since every translation is historically situated: "when we choose a word to translate it, we tilt each passage with a particular load of *psuchē*'s semantic heritage, picking over the debris from centuries of reflection accumulated between the early Greeks and ourselves" (Padel 1992, 32).

The third term of the triad, *nous*, or "mind" seen as intellect, the thinking ability, is unlike either *thōmos* or *psuchē* in that it has no ethnolocation within the body as such. *Nous*, in fact, functions in a way similar to the Melpa *noman*, of which people say that of course you could not see it if you cut open the chest of a person. *Nous* can be hidden, just as *noman* is in Melpa, and the idea that it is "in the body" expresses this characteristic. You cannot look into it, *just as* you cannot look into a person's insides. *Nous* seems to operate in the same fashion as, and parallel to, organs and thus gains a kind of "concreteness" (33). It also assimilates persons to the divine, or, as Euripides suggested, "*Nous* is to us in each of us a god," an idea with a distinct resemblance to Descartes's idea of the intellect as that portion of us which is akin to God.

Rightly, Padel cautions against too easy an appeal to our own ideas of metaphor, constructed *against* ideas of the literal or real, in interpreting ancient Greek expressions. She points to the holistic quality of Greek thought, shared by many others, such as the Ilongot or the Melpa. Yet she warns also against too concrete a form of interpretation, referring instead to a "somatic tinge" in meanings and suggesting that such meanings may have been nuanced and complex from early times onward (Padel 1992, 36, 38). Nevertheless, she recognizes the strength of the "somatic model," as it were, acknowledging that many of the words she discusses "seem (to us at least) to pull this concreteness into their own behavioral range" (39). She warns further against too easy a decision that expressions are either literal or metaphorical, since this distinction itself belongs to our own worldview and not necessarily to that of other people (see A. J. Strathern 1993a). "It is not useful," she says, "to project semantic fields of our own words, like heart, soul, mind, or spirit, or to talk in terms of slippage" (Padel 1992, 39).

One key to the Greek ideas appears to lie precisely in the question of the relationship between the insides of the body and the outside world. The channels hypothesized by different peoples in this regard often constitute their "psychology" or their "religion" or, equally, their "science" in our terms. By the late fifth century B.C. in Greece this communication between outside and inside was thought predominantly to take place through *poroi* (cf. English *pores*). And the communication was held to be facilitated by the fact that human bodies are made of the same stuff as the world they inhabit. Hence the theory of the "elements" (earth, water, air, and fire) and the humors of the body (blood, water, black bile, and yellow bile). Since these elements, as we have already seen for blood and bile, carried moral (and therefore, for us, mental) characteristics, it is clear that for the Greeks of this period also the body was seen directly as mindful. Padel quotes a passage in Parmenides that expresses the idea that *noos* (= *nous*), or mind, is present in all the limbs of the body: an idea that finds a parallel in the Wiru culture of Pangia in Papua New Guinea in which *wene* (mind, will, intention) is held to inhere in both limbs and organs including the genitals, so that a woman's vagina, for example, has its own *wene,* and the male penis is conceptualized as an actor on its own behalf: *tekene tuku toa wakome andene lingako* (searching in vain for a vagina, the penis stands up stiff [or *nengako,* "stands up *very* stiff"]).

Humoral ideas were, of course, systematized in the Hippocratic corpus of writings on medicine, which combined an apparently rigorous materialism with an appropriation of basic elements that were either linked to divinity or held to be influenced by divinity in popular culture. The Hippocratic exercise was thus in a sense like that of Descartes much later: the creation of a sphere for "rational science" by means of a disguised preservation of religious ideas. Whether this is an entirely accurate characterization of the intentions of either the Hippocratic writers or of Descartes, it does, I believe, capture an aspect of the effects they had on subsequent thought and particularly of the "intellectual space" that they created. With Hippocratic medicine the pathway toward biomedicine was opened up. Closed in certain regards by Christian dogmas in medieval times, it was reopened by Descartes with his mechanistic-materialistic view of causation within the body. But Hippocratic medicine, I am arguing, covertly contained religious elements via the sacred character of the elements and the receptiveness of humors in the body to these elements.

Outside of the Hippocratic tradition this same worldview underpinned a complex of ideas regarding illness and divination, to which Padel refers in the second and third chapters of her book. She points out that the Hippocratic writers incorporated aspects of this tradition into their own texts, and presumably they did this in order to obtain clients for their practices. A belief in the influence of seasonal changes on the human body links the old (religious) and the new (materialist-secular) views together. There was a discourse also that linked epidemics to civil war, as also one that compared erotic desire to disease (consider our word *lovesick*). "Illness in the Greek thought-world is inseparable from passion or pollution" (Padel 1992, 54).

Consistently, with such ideas that disease enters the body from the outside and causes illness, therapeutic medicine stressed the eviction of pathogenic elements by means of bloodletting, sweating, draining, etc., the purging of substances that are not in a balanced state (e.g., between hot and cold) (Padel 1992, 55). Those organs that communicate with the outside world were especially involved in the transmission of disease, including the eyes (hence the concept of the evil eye). Oedipus blinded himself so as to stop the "two-way traffic" between himself and the world (63).

The innards of the human body, which were thought of as becoming "darkened" by strong emotions, illness, or madness, were also regarded as repositories of divinatory truth, an idea expressed in Aeschylus' play *Agamemnon*: "the innards *(splanchna)* do not speak in vain, heart circling beside the truthful *phrenes* in prophetic spirals" (Padel 1992, 73). Another source of insight came from dreams, especially those of seers who slept in caves. There seems to be an analogy here between the innards within the body and the seer within the cave, a kind of fractal replication of the same structure at different scales of being. Such a fractal factor probably underlies all humoral systems of medicine, in fact, and corresponds further to Bourdieu's definition of the habitus as a "durable, *transposable* disposition" (my emph.).

The idea that disturbances enter the body from outside itself entered into gendered definitions of processes of possession by the gods. As Padel notes, "one concrete image for the relation between a possessing god and the mind is erotic penetration of female by male" (1992, 106). Such an image schema particularly underlay the cult of Apollo at Delphi, where the Pythian priestess was supposed to be both unmarried and to be entered by the god through the open parts of her body (Sissa 1990). As a vessel, then, mind was envisaged in a female manner, whereas mind as agent was envisaged as male. From such an equation issues, of course, a long tradition of "phallocentric" thought in European cultures. Yet female passivity could also be creative. It could "nourish" thought, and it could be "pregnant" already from its own internal power. Or it could be a source of passion and danger. As Padel notes, "It is consciously important to Greek thought that what is destructive may also illuminate" (1992,113). Fifth-century Athenian society was male dominated, and women were conceptualized as creatures of the house, of the inside, of darkness, creative but also in some senses threatening. The conceptualizations of the body that accompanied such ideas flowed later into Christianity also, although the tenor of morality in Christianity was quite different from that in earlier Greek culture, as Foucault urges in his *History of Sexuality* (1990). Gendered ideas about the mind, and thus its relationship to the body, persisted also in theological and philosophical writings from Plato onward, through Aristotle, Philo, Saint Augustine, and Thomas Aquinas (Lloyd 1984, 19–37).

Peter Brown, in his detailed study *The Body and Society* (1988), has traced many of the pathways of historical influence that led into the Middle Ages via the Greco-Roman world. He notes the fundamental opposition between Roman civic ideas of the necessity to reproduce in order to remain politically strong and Christian ideas of sexual renunciation. From the idea of the virgin birth of Jesus and the model of divine (male) purity that sustains it through to Saint Paul's elevation of celibacy as an ideal coupled with his dry recognition that some will need to marry because "it is better to marry than to burn" (with desire? or in Hell? perhaps both?), it is evident that Christianity gathered into

itself a mode of thinking about sexuality that cannot be exactly paralleled in pre-Christian Greek or Roman culture. Nor does it equate with
Jewish culture, although the idea of male (or female) ascetic purity and
celibacy as a condition for having prophetic powers was present in
both Jewish and pagan cultures prior to Christianity (Brown 1988, 67;
see also Sissa 1990). A male-dominated church headed by senior celibate males attended also by senior celibate females gave a bodily representation of such values and ensured a spiritual hierarchy between
"the church" and "the world" that still contributes to the authority of
the pope vis-à-vis Catholic congregations around the world.

In Christian thinking sexual purity, attainable in principle only
through celibacy, became the supreme sign of spiritual purity, a renunciation of the world and the flesh in favor of the spirit and the light of
God. In keeping with aspects of the Greek tradition, erotic desire was
seen as an aberration, and it was associated also with that which was
female. By inciting male lust, female bodies become themselves culpa-
ble, a mark of the flesh and of sin, of death and darkness as against resurrection and light. "The serpent deceived me, and I did eat" associated
Eve with a cthonian power that in Greek traditions was in fact a source
of fertility and renewal but in Judaic tradition became the incarnation
of evil (Sanday 1981, 224 ff., and her further suggestions, in addition to
my own here, that both serpent and tree were sacred symbols in ancient
Canaanite religion and that ritual sex with temple prostitutes may be a
covert theme underlying the Genesis story).

The value placed on sexual continence obviously created a divided
self and an ambivalence toward the body as the source of temptation.
As Peter Brown puts it (1988, 108), "The . . . human person mirrored,
with terrible precision, the confusion that lay at the root of the physical
universe. The body was deeply alien to the true self. It was not simply
an inferior other that might be brought to order by the vigorous soul"
(as in the pagan Greek ideal of becoming *basileus heautou*, "king of oneself," a model of centralized control over unruly parts). Brown is here
describing the teachings of the Gnostic Valentinus in the second century A.D., in whose scheme "even the soul, the *psyché [psuchē]* the conscious self, had occurred as an afterthought . . . [and] swathed the lucid
spirit in a thick fog of doubt, anxiety and passion." Valentinus' scheme
of thought was simply one version of the general Christian devaluation
of sexuality as such, carried to the length of supposing there to be a
pure spirit beyond the *psuchē,* which was seen as entangled in mortal

emotions (as it would be, since the concept had earlier absorbed the characteristics formerly attributed to the *thūmos*).

If we move forward to the fourth and fifth centuries A.D. and consider the work of Saint Augustine of Hippo, we can project the account into the early Middle Ages from that point. Augustine in his *Confessions* presents the same picture of sexuality as Valentinus and, in harmony with the Greek traditions idealized by Plato, he praises intellectual friendship between males and places it above the pleasures of heterosexual intercourse and thus is led to extol the idea of a church formed of a continent male elite (Brown 1988, 391). The Manichaeans, contemporary with Augustine, took this position further: sexuality itself was evil, and the body should be subjugated by ascetic starvation so as to empty it of desire. Related to this theme is that of the mortification of the senses, a deliberately adopted *askesis,* which Augustine explicitly describes (see Burke 1961, 138–41). Phenomena of this kind show the force of Foucault's approach to history through the body (see, e.g., Foucault 1990). Augustine acquainted himself with Manichaean teachings, and later with the Neoplatonist writings of Plotinus and Porphyry, which inspired him to a mystical vision of spiritual delight or pleasure, an event that led him further to devalue sexuality as such, even though his own images of his vision take on a distinctly sexual cast. After he became a Catholic bishop, "Augustine moved in a monochrome, all-male world" (Brown 1988, 396), but he also created a theology that was compatible with the Roman Empire that was necessary as the vehicle for the continuity of the Catholic Church. In this theology Adam and Eve were reconstituted as the prototype of the properly married pair, and thus sexuality was allowed as the cornerstone of the family.

Augustine also envisaged friendship between a married pair as enduring beyond their period of sexual activity. The problem he identified for humanity was not simply the original fall from grace and the identification of that fall with knowledge of sexuality but, rather, the perversions of sexuality that humans invented and the thoughts of it that continued to follow Augustine himself into his later years, producing in him the sensation of a divided self (Brown 1988, 407). Such a distressing awareness of sex was, he said, a *discordiosum malum,* "an abiding principle of discord lodged in the human person since the Fall" (408). It revealed a *concupiscentia carnis,* a bodily desire that tilted persons towards the flesh (418) but was, in fact, the product of a distorted soul. Augustine essentialized and dramatized the problem of sexuality in ways that fed into medieval ideas (even though his doctrines were opposed by Julian, a bishop of Eclanum in southern Italy). Simply by pointing to the existential dangers of sexuality, Augustine had also "placed sexuality irremovably at the center of the human person" (422). The body and its sexuality were a problem simply because Augustine saw it as something not to be abused but cared for. His ideal (expressed in male language and revealing the same gender categories as we have noted earlier) was that "Your flesh is like your wife. . . . Love it, rebuke it; let it be formed into one bond of body and soul" (426). Yet the image of marriage contained within it a sense of perpetual discord as well as an ideal of harmony. Implicitly also in Augustine's formulation the self is seen as the mind and as male, married to a body that is in a sense female. It is, of course, the same image that informed the supposed relationship between God and his church. Yet this male power could not guarantee peace because of its own internal division. Hence Augustine's question "When will full peace come to even one single person?" Brown neatly sums up the effect of Augustine's work as the creation of a "darkened humanism," a suitable prelude in a way to the overall gloomy views of humanity that dominated the later ages.

The views of Augustine were, however, not as extreme in themselves as those of the Neoplatonist Gnostics. While Augustine saw the body as an object to be loved, the Gnostics thought of it as a prison from which the soul longed to escape through *gnosis*, "knowledge" (Williams 1989, 129). Gnostic ideas thus form one ascetic and theological basis for monkhood and nunhood in the Christian church. Gnostic teachings distinguished between the psychic body, or soul body, first created by the deity and the physical body created secondarily, hence the image of a "soul" entombed within flesh, as a body itself is wrapped in a garment of cloth. Only the upright human posture was considered beautiful and a mark of distinction by contrast with animals. The head and its brain were considered images of male power, in line with other, much older traditions in Greek culture. And Williams points out that, while they in a sense devalued the body, the Gnostics were intrigued by it as a kind of model, so that "truths, both pleasant and unpleasant, about their origin and their destiny could be traced within its form and functions" (143).

In Catholic Christianity a similar fascination with the body— for one thing, in later medieval times it was seen as the material for eventual resurrection—came to center on the Body of Christ as the Savior of mankind. One concern was with the face of Christ and the division of opinion between the Eastern and Western churches (Baudinet 1989). This has to do with different representations of authority. But another theme relates the Body of Christ to the female body (Bynum 1989). Bynum's study centers on the later Middle Ages, the thirteenth century onward. Bynum's work takes up themes of gender classifications noted by Padel in her study of pre-Christian Greek culture. Like Padel also, she argues that classifications and ideas were more complex than is sometimes allowed. Christian dogma emphasized patriarchy and the dangers of sexuality and the body, identified with the female. Yet this same identification came to lend a strongly somatic quality to the spirituality of medieval women. Her argument, in fact, suggests a kind of "comeback of the body" at this time, prefiguring later transformations (see also Bynum 1994). Perhaps she is also describing elements in popular culture that had existed all along, unnoticed in the tracts of bishops.

First, she notes the prevalent use of bodily relics and also substances as sources of power—for example, breast milk from holy virgins (Bynum 1994, 163). Self-torture of the body was used by saints to chastise themselves but also to achieve a union of their bodies with that of Jesus and his sufferings. Female mystics described the process with erotic overtones (much as Augustine described his spiritual visions and desires). Communion also became more "bodily" in ethos: the consumption of the power of Jesus. Oral themes are also exhibited in relation to Christ's foreskin, which one mystic declared she had received "in her mouth in a vision and found it to taste as sweet as honey" (164). (Similar erotic themes can be found in contemporary Pentecostal hymns sung by strongly female congregations in Papua New Guinea: themes of falling in love with Jesus so that "He gets sweeter as the days go by / Oh, what a joy between my Lord and I!")

Such bodily images and their associations with the female appear to have increased in Europe from the twelfth century onward. Especially female mystics became subject to trance, levitations, and seizures as well as an inability to consume anything but the eucharistic host ("holy anorexia") (Bynum 1994, 165). Female mystics exuded sweet mucus from their necks or sweet-smelling oil from their bodies at death, and their bodies were said not to decay. Their illnesses frequently were accounted to be a part of their marks of sanctity, and some prayed for such illness "as a gift from God" (166). Illness was therefore cherished rather than cured, again especially in women rather than men. Further, participation in Christ's body is a female theme. "Women regularly speak of tasting God, of kissing Him deeply, of going into his heart or entrails, of being covered by His blood." One poetess and mystic spoke of embracing Christ until "all my members felt his full felicity" (168). The bodily image of Christ is necessary to such visions and experiences, as is the idea of a soul that is not separate from the body but is, rather, "a creature who is the life of the flesh" (170).

Bynum asks why this theme of the female mystical body emerged at this time. It is seen as female empowerment and a justification of the (sanctified) flesh as something good. The experiential quality of women's writings is due to the fact that they expressed themselves in the vernacular, not having access to Church Latin—but the idea of women as representing the bodily side of experience is, as we have seen, much older than this time, reaching back into early Greek culture. This bodily side had itself two aspects: the flesh as evil, mortal, or the flesh as a source of positive mystical experience. Misogynist conclusions were drawn from the "evil" aspect, but the female body was also (and somewhat paradoxically) associated with the human aspect of Christ. Christ's own body and his wounds are often given a female aspect, as though the wounds, for example, imitated the female action of menstruating from the vagina. Such an idea derived from the basic identification of the church, seen as female, with Christ's body. Christ was understood as a duality, his divine aspect male, his human aspect female, marked also by the pure body of his mother, Mary. Such a theory chimed in with the Aristotelian doctrine that in reproduction the male provided the form while the female provided substance (i.e., flesh, body). While such a dogma elevated males, it gave to women a special connection with the body, just as Christian doctrine did.

Bynum further argues that in the later Middle Ages theorists came to see body and soul as joined together in a unity (i.e., rejection of Neoplatonism and strong dualism). The body-soul distinction was frequently subverted "either by inserting entities between body and soul or by obscuring their differences" (Bynum 1994, 188–89). Interests in miracles, possession, and medical questions all centered on the body. Resurrection was at issue also, with the idea that, while the soul survives death, it will be reunited with the resurrected body at the end of time in order to form the full human being *(totus homo)*. The soul here is the anima (192; citing Thomas Aquinas). With Aquinas's idea that soul and body are one being, it follows that the soul is affected by bodily suffering (and vice versa, incidentally). For mystics of this time Augustine's attitude to the body was revivified: "source of temptation and torment, it is also a beloved companion and helpmeet" (197). (Cf. the expression *hospes comesque corporis* in the words of the Emperor Hadrian.)

These late medieval theories, practices, and experiences show us not only the reworking of ancient ideas and their fluctuations in Christian history but also the legacy of theological-philosophical problems that they passed on in a modified and complex manner and that formed the background to Descartes's thinking, which I suggested at the beginning of this chapter should be found if we are to see to what extent he innovated, and to what extent he followed, cultural categories developed before him. Another point is also clear: it is the soul, not the mind, that was the focus of concern in medieval times, and this soul was in intimate union with the body. Descartes's scheme therefore represents a break with that tradition, an intellectualist position that was theologically convenient but also fell—interestingly enough—to the strictures of a female critic, Elizabeth of Bohemia, on just those grounds of the union between soul and body that had been formulated in the theology of Thomas Aquinas. Such a "psychosomatic" picture of the person, as Bynum labels it, is in fact quite similar to the picture of the mindful body that now replaces Descartes's separatist schemes of thought in medical anthropology.

The psychosomatic picture of the body and sickness owes, of course, a great deal to the work of Sigmund Freud. Although I do not in this book attempt any serious consideration of Freud's work, it is important to notice that his interests in the "motivated" character of physical disorders and their sources in trauma and repression definitely contributed to the formation of concepts that have subsequently appeared in anthropology as "somatization" (e.g., in the work of Alfred Kleinman; see also Kleinman 1988, for a rethinking of these issues). With the theory of repression Freud intended to build an idea of the unconscious mind, but his implication is that this mind also shows itself in bodily patterns of behavior of which the conscious mind may not be aware or which it cannot control. Freud also saw many of the original sources of behavior in the powerful early bodily experiences of the child (breastfeeding as unconditional love; anality as an interest in feces to be banished by socialization and repressed; the oral, anal, and genital phases of sexuality, etc.). He further argued that patterns of association emerging into forms of fantasy and symbolism depended first on repression and then the displacement, condensation, and reversibility of meanings: one form of displacement, indeed, being "into the body." The body thus becomes the site of unconscious, socialized meanings, as it does later in Pierre Bourdieu's scheme, but with the additional theory of repression as the fundamental mechanism whereby such meanings are driven into the body in this way. Finally, Freud's theory of the body is highly gendered, not only because of his stress on sexual repression (derivable from his own patriarchal milieu, perhaps) but also because of his specific hypothesis of the Oedipus complex, the importance of the penis and the fear of castration (for latter-day Lacanian lucubrations on this theme, see Baudrillard 1993). Both condensation and displacement are hypothesized, for example, in his suggestion of a symbolic equation between penis and baby. Freud's theories have often been taken up by anthropologists in their quest for "meanings" of practices, whether with or without his own historicist modes of explanation (for a recent ethnography that uses a Freudian approach, see Gillison 1993; although Freud is mentioned only on p. 49, his influence seems pervasive in this work). A lighthearted but also serious evaluation of Freud's work on "the symbolic" is given also by Kenneth Burke (see, e.g., 1961, 260–65; 1966, 63–80; 1973, 258–92,) and see also Wallace 1983, for a general consideration of Freud and anthropology.

As I have suggested in passing more than once, the kinds of ideas about the body that are found in cultures of the Pacific—and in many other parts of the world—are closer to a "psychosomatic" model also than they are to a Cartesian dualistic scheme. It is to a more extended consideration of these Pacific cultures that I turn next, bearing in mind both the "intellectual baggage" that outsiders have inevitably brought to the study of these cultures and the warnings by Ruth Padel against ethnocentric projections in the translation of terms.

Chapter 4

The Becoming Body

Accounts of the body in Melanesian cultures have tended to focus on life cycle processes and their underpinnings in local theories regarding conception, growth, nutrition, health, sickness, maturity, and decline. It is a valuable approach, and one that helped to shift the study of initiation practices, for example, away from modes of interpretation based on Western psychological theories and toward a deeper understanding of the peoples' own concepts, ideologies, and rationales. This particular focus, also, has given us a new way of considering the operation of kinship systems and the constructions of personhood found in Melanesia. The element of agency, however, and its analytical marker, the mindful body, tend to be somewhat left aside in these analyses. Yet, if we put such "substance-oriented" analyses together with "agency-oriented" discussions, the effect will be to enrich further our understanding of both personhood and individuality in these cultures.

In this chapter I will explore this point, using as loci for the discussion some recurrent themes that appear in the ethnography: blood and pollution; conception and procreation theories, and theories of death, the life cycle, life force, and the mind; the skin and its capacities; and, finally, historical changes in ideas regarding the body resulting from the impact of introduced forms of clothing.

One aspect of the data needs to be emphasized at the outset: we are dealing with ideas that among other things, form an indigenous aesthetics as well as a morality or a rationale for, say, exchange practices. Practices to do with the body are often aimed at enhancing its appeal and attractiveness, and they celebrate the power of that appeal in social relationships. "The Becoming Body," my chapter title, is intended to convey both the sense of the body involved in change over the life cycle and the sense of the body as good, desirable, suitable. What we find is that the good condition of the body is never aimed at in isolation from other actions and values but always in conjunction with these. The body is thus, as Mary Douglas argued, a vehicle for the expression of such values (see also Gell 1993, on Polynesian tattooing).

Bruce Knauft, in his erudite and stimulating survey article "Bodily Images in Melanesia: Cultural Substances and Natural Metaphors" (1989), has performed a valuable service by pulling together many references to the body and its substances in Melanesia. He has also drawn attention to the significance of costuming as a "primary art form in the region," "with a diversity and beauty of decoration matched by the intricacy of local spiritual symbolism" (200). The ideal body thus created is also one that is "defined fundamentally through social and spiritual relationships," he writes (201). He therefore begins by negating individualistic concepts of the body and the self that are a part of Western culture. In this he is right: myriad examples show that the thoughts and attitudes and actions of kinsfolk, living and dead, are held to influence the health of the person, and therefore the body as the site of health or sickness is also the site of socially defined and constrained morality. It is important to stress that this is exactly what is negated in principle by biomedicine, which treats sickness as physical and therefore morally neutral (see Conrad and Schneider 1992). Such a proposition can work only in a tradition that has inherited a Cartesian separation between body and mind. In Melanesian cultural thinking conditions are certainly physical, but the physical is intimately tied to the mental and the social. Physical conditions are considered to be the *results* of mental and social factors, and the curing of sickness therefore depends on tracking down such factors and dealing with them. These factors, however, are an outcome of people's *choices* to think and do certain things. Therefore, agency, if not individuality, must be taken into account if we wish to understand how the cycle of events is conceived of by the people. Knauft has made this same point, but he phrases it in a more collectively oriented fashion, thus: "self and body are transactionally constituted through social relationships and through belief in spiritual forces" (203). He proceeds, therefore, to examine ideas about the body in the framework of life cycle processes. My treatment of topics will be in counterpoint with his: I do not use the life cycle as such as an organizing framework, but the topics I choose would have their place in such a framework. I begin with theories of pollution.

Pollution, Fertility, and Power

I have discussed earlier (chap. 1) Mary Douglas's ideas on pollution. These really fall into two parts, general and specific. Parker has summarized the general versions of her ideas quite well: (1) "a society may use a supposed physical impurity as an unconscious symbol upon which it focuses fears and concerns of a much broader social character" and (2) "pollution is in general a property of the betwixt and between; that which falls between or violates the categories into which a given society divides external reality is accounted by that society impure" (Parker 1983, 56, 61). The first formulation stresses emotions and the unconscious; the second speaks to logic and structural viewpoint. In the specific applications of her ideas Douglas argued that the body acts as a symbol of dangers to group boundaries or to the organization of control over and between persons in social networks. Agency is omitted from this perspective or rather agency is attributed, as in Parker's rendition, to "society," instead of to individual actors or to ideologically motivated categories of actors (such as "dominant males"). We are left also to exercise choice in deciding *what* the dangers are that are being symbolized. One such danger is "pressure on external boundaries," of course, and in the spirit of such an approach, Mervyn Meggitt argued for the Mae Enga people of the Papua New Guinea Highlands that fear of menstrual pollution is a reflection (unconscious?) of the fear of attack by enemies, since men marry wives from enemy groups (Meggitt 1964; see also Brown and Buchbinder 1976). Such wives, who move from their natal areas to live with their husbands, can also be seen as "betwixt and between," ambiguous categories subject ex hypothesi to being considered as taboo, or polluting, in certain respects.

Several questions, of course, arise out of this mode of analysis. First, male *ideas* regarding the powers of female menstrual blood share features across a considerable variety of social structural settings. They are not confined to cases in which affines are enemies (see chap. 1). Second, given the point that women are seen as betwixt and between, we still have to explain why menstruation, and not some other feature of their being, becomes a focus of male anxiety (an ad hoc recourse to Freudian theory could here be made). Third, we can ask how precisely does the social logic involved operate? If we ask this question we can, in fact, drive a pathway through the difficulties in analysis.

There is perhaps no need to hypothesize an unconscious, societal locus for male fear and anxiety, since the ethnotheories of the people themselves satisfactorily explain, at a perfectly conscious level, what these fears are about. (We could argue, of course, that unconscious factors are also at work.) Danger comes to the male body through contact with female blood, either at the time of menstruation or subsequently, since pieces of blood are held to stick onto and inside the vagina. Men's skins will lose their glossy appearance and become dull and ashen colored; they themselves will grow thin; the menstrual blood will rise to their throats through their penises and choke them. This ever-present anxiety, based on ideas that are widely spread, is then intensified in those societies in which women from enemy groups are often married. These women may owe loyalty still to their natal kin, who may wish to kill the husbands in revenge for past killings in either warfare or sorcery attacks. In Melpa society it is said that women may be ensorcelled by their male natal kin (made "crazy," [wulya wulya] by magic that turns their *noman,* or mind, around) and thus persuaded to kill their husband either with their own menstrual blood or with another form of "poison" that they are given to administer. All of these scenarios, therefore, invoke agency as well as structure. The fear of menstrual blood is not, perhaps, fully explained but the pragmatic contexts of such fear are elucidated, and it is ethnotheories of the body that are in focus rather than imputed depth psychologies.

Buckley and Gottlieb (1988) have criticized "reductionistic theoretical frameworks" used to explain ideas about menstruation. They note the virtues of a biocultural approach and argue that a stress on "menstrual taboos" is misplaced. Menstruation is a more complex phenomenon, and its meanings are more multivalent than is allowed by the taboo formulation. They rebut the general theory that menstrual taboos are simply used to oppress women (9 ff.), as also the appeal to the idea that menstrual taboos are based on forms of neurosis (15). They also reject the literality of theories that argue that menstrual blood is *actually* dangerous to men (through the presence of menotoxins) or that some game animals are *actually* repelled by menstrual odors (19: here they are commenting on the explanation of taboos, common enough among hunting peoples, on having sex and on being around menstruating women when a hunting expedition is at hand; see also Knight 1991, and note that women's sexual parts are *also* held by some peoples to attract game). Instead, they argue for a holistic approach. We must understand menstrual symbolism fully before we attempt to explain it: no etics without prior emics.

Utilizing Mary Douglas's phrase that "dirt is matter out of place," they first consider menstruation as blood outside of its proper "place," the body, and therefore as potentially dangerous or polluting. They correctly point out that menstrual blood has to be compared with other discharges of blood that are equally "out of place." Menstrual blood has a special significance since it signifies reproductive power and has a potentially positive valency in this regard rather than simply a negative polluting capacity. Menstrual discharges are liminal and therefore powerful in relation to either life or death. Gottlieb and Buckley quote an "ethnographically informed rendering" of a conversation from S. Illinois to the effect that, if a woman put menstrual blood in her husband's coffee, she would retain his love. (A similar idea holds in Pangia in the Southern Highlands of Papua New Guinea, where it is held that small pieces of vaginal hair clippings can have the same effect.) As they note, examples of this sort point to an ethnotheory of shared substance rather than to a concept of pollution, and they suggest that a dialectic of positive and negative poles in relation to menstrual blood is probably more common than has been allowed. The terms of earlier debates about "pollution" only were therefore misplaced.

Buckley and Gottlieb, in what is perhaps their most interesting move, go on to argue that attitudes about menstrual blood may depend on ethnotheories of conception: "we hypothesize that where the fetus is held to be menstrually constituted, one will find strong menstrual taboos" (1988, 39). They quote the case of the Paiela of Papua New Guinea (Biersack 1983), whose views on this matter duplicate those of the Melpa people—namely, that conception occurs when amounts of semen are able, as a result of repeated acts of intercourse, to bind the blood in a woman's womb and so form a fetus. Discharge of such blood is therefore a loss, a failure of reproduction, a kind of "miscarriage." While the blood may be in a sense polluting, its discharge may also be a purification that is held to conduce toward further sexual and reproductive activity.

Lifting their analysis to a more general level, Buckley and Gottlieb reach conclusions that are exactly in line with the theme of the mindful body. They argue that the meaning of menstrual symbolism must be grounded in ethnobiological theories, on the one hand, and in the dialectic of body and mind as this is perceived cross-culturally on the other. They add that it is *our* (Western) separation of body and mind that makes it hard for us to perceive this point. We try to read either from society to body (as Mary Douglas does) or from body to society (as the sociobiologists do), rather than understanding that the relationship is a dialectical one, *mediated by mind,* and therefore by agency and experience as well as by formal cultural constructions. Implicitly, they suggest that the search for purely sociological explanations is unlikely to be successful. At the least, there is the tertium quid of ethnobiology to take into account.

Further attention to some New Guinea examples will enable us to follow up Buckley and Gottlieb's various insights. First, there is the point that menstrual blood is *blood,* in a certain state or phase. It may especially signify female reproductive power, but blood generally, and for both sexes, carries connotations in many cultures of power, vitality, life, life force. Among the Melpa, if blood is shed from a wound, it must be fixed or fastened again by an immediate compensation payment of wealth goods, which is seen as the equivalent of the blood itself. This is called *mema pendenemen* (they make to be the blood [i.e., put it back, restore it]). Without this payment the wound will not heal, because the wounded person is still *ararimb* (angry) as a result of not being offered the payment itself (see A. J. Strathern n.d.). The immediate payment thus has a therapeutic function, to help the victim's body heal, expressed as "fixing the blood." In Pangia the sight of blood flowing from a wound can also be disturbing to the viewer: in 1967 I once had to pay a small compensation to an old man, Longai, who had noticed blood coming from a scratch on my leg. The logic here is that the viewer's sympathy for the other diminishes his own blood, which should then be restored with a payment. For the Gnau people of the West Sepik in Papua New Guinea the penile blood of a *wauwi* (mother's brother) is important in the initiation ritual of his sister's son. It is cooked with the special stew, *wa'agep,* which is fed to the boy to strengthen him, while at the same time his skin is smeared with red betel juice, a substance that is also imbued with life force (Lewis 1980, 73–74, 77, 174). In this case there is no mediation with wealth, but blood itself is given as a prestation between kin, as a transmission of positive male life force.

Among the Paiela menstruating women make magic to ensure the beauty of their husbands, and this magic is presided over by a female spirit, the "ginger-woman" (Biersack 1982, 242). The same spirit is held to be involved in assisting the growth of adolescent boys, through what Biersack calls an "occult equivalent of simple nurturance" (241), directed toward the increase of fat or juice under the skin (the Paiela term *ipane* derives from the word for "water"). This process is invisible and is said to occur secretly at night and as a result of magical force, ultimately dependent on the moon, which is imaged as the sister of the male sun. The growth of adolescent boys takes place in a peripheral cult location within the forest, where they are spoken of as married to the female spirit. They avoid eating foods that would make their skin "small" and "dull," and they must not be seen by adults who are living a life of actual sexual intercourse. Their seclusion is therefore purificatory. A ritual wash in a spring near to the cult enclosure contributes to their cleansing by removing from their eyes the "filthy" things they have seen. (These parts of the ritual are comparable to those reported for the Mae Enga to the east of the Paicla [Meggitt 1964]. They remove their ordinary clothing and dress in bush materials, hoping that the ginger-woman will take pity on them and come to "sit in their skins" and so make them grow (Biersack 1982, 245). Under the tutelage of a senior bachelor, who is spoken of as "giving" the spirit woman to the boys as a "bride" in return for the wealth that they pay to him, they plant ginger roots in an act that is held to stimulate the growth of their own head hair (equated with ginger in terms of its regenerative capacities). They also place bamboo tubes in swampy places and later check these to see if the water that has seeped into them is clear and plentiful. If so, this is a sign that the ginger-woman is not menstruating and is growing the inner skin of the boys. The boys eventually emerge, decked with forest finery, and perform a *mali* dance in the settlement place before the eyes of the adult people. Pork fat rubbed on their chests is said to gleam as a result of the presence of the ginger-woman.

As Biersack demonstrates, a binary code of oppositions underlies these ritual activities, with a set of parallel contrasts between peripheral/place central place; secrecy/publicity; magical, invisible growth/visible embodied display; and purification/defilement. The ginger-woman also operates in a way that inverts the sexual relations between human couples. She has a name "but no body," and her act of inducing growth in the boys takes place when she is not menstruating, whereas married human women make growth or beauty magic for their husbands while they are menstruating.

Biersack further explains that a married Paiela women can express her good or bad intentions toward her husband at the time of her menstruation. If she is angry with him, she may not bother to do the magic, or she may do it so as to spoil the husband's "skin" (Biersack 1982, 242). As with all her data, it is remarkable here how the Paiela stress intentionality and choice. The ginger-woman also expresses her intentions by helping or not helping the boys to grow. The Paiela concept of *nembo* (equivalent to Melpa *noman*, "mind") underlies this. Paiela bodies are thus, by definition, linked to mind: actions are mindful, and the body (skin) is a result of these actions; it embodies mind.

This example of the use of menstrual blood for growth or beauty magic may be surprising, given the usual Highlands ideology that menstrual blood spoils men's skins, essentially by removing their fat and making them dry. Perhaps Paiela women's ritual actions are apotropaic: they may be neutralizing the putative harmful quality of their menstrual blood. Yet there is evidence from two other areas not far from the Paiela that suggests menstrual blood can have a positive aspect in *ritual* contexts. Among the Duna people, who belong to a language area that abuts on western Paiela territory, there was in the past a special ritual that involved the taking of the menstrual blood of an unmarried girl on a journey to a sacred site in Huli territory to the south, Kelote, and its offering to spirits in the earth as a means of appeasing them and ensuring fertility (Stürzenhofecker 1995). And among the Baktaman and Telefolmin, who live further west of the Duna, Maureen Mackenzie reports that *gagan isak*, a ceremonial red paint used to decorate young male initiates, consists of red ocher from a sacred site, believed to "represent [the mythical creative female spirit] Afek's generative and nurturant blood" (Mackenzie 1991, 179), and also of real menstrual blood obtained in cooperation with the women who produce it. While men generally stress the importance of pig fat (seen as a male substance perhaps analogous to semen) in causing growth of the novitiates, this use of red ocher and blood clearly indicates the complementarity of the sexes at a most fundamental level. Mackenzie's data, supported by those gathered by Jorgensen (1981, 395; qtd. in Mackenzie 1991, 179), are all the more striking because her points about menstrual blood and the color of red ocher are not to be found in Poole's accounts of Bimin-Kuskusmin initiation (Poole 1982) or in Fredrik Barth's work on the Baktaman (Barth 1975). Barth in fact stresses that the color red is associated with male ancestors (77), and he describes acts of painting initiates with red mixtures reminiscent of those recounted by Mackenzie: fourth-degree initiates are painted with a mixture of pork fat, red pandanus juice, and a red tree juice, the aim being to color their whole bodies a brilliant red (74). If, nevertheless, female elements are covertly introduced into the paint mixture, it is possible that Barth's informants did not mention this, following practices of concealment that are common in cultures of the Ok region, where the Baktaman live. A formal male ideology that menstrual blood is polluting and dangerous seems thus to be secretly countermanded in ritual practices that reveal instead the recognition that the sexes are interdependent. Perhaps it is the *mixture* of male and female elements that confers the magical power on the paint used to enhance the skins (visible bodies) of the initiates. This formulation would enable us to argue that "male" and "female" powers are admitted not to work alone or in isolation; indeed, by themselves and when "out of place" they can be dangerous and destructive. When combined ritually, however, and harnessed by male control as well as female cooperation, they produce fertility. The same logic applies to Melpa ritual actions centered on stones of the *Amb Kor,* a female spirit. These stones are rubbed with pork fat and red ocher before being wrapped in moss and buried (as semen and blood are wrapped in the womb to produce a child). (See also Bonnemère 1992, on pandanus juice among the Ankave people of Eastern Highlands Province.)

This point returns us to Buckley and Gottlieb's proposition regarding conception theories. The idea that semen binds the blood and therefore forms an encompassing container for it is an aspect of male-oriented ideology that goes with gender hierarchy in many of the New Guinea Highlands cultures. The Daribi people have an elaborate set of ideas based on the same "container" or "binding," image as the Melpa (see also LiPuma 1988, 42, on Maring ideas). "The semen then forms the external parts of the body, the skin, muscle tissue, toenails, fingernails, teeth, eyes, and hair, while the mother's blood forms the blood and bones, and the liver, lungs, heart, stomach, intestines, and other internal organs" (Wagner 1967, 64). The mother's blood, *page-kamine,* is that of her own brother and hence the father must make payments for this, to secure the child's affiliation, a fact that indicates that blood represents as strong a claim as semen, unless it is "bought off" (compensated for) with vital wealth. Semen gives the right to claim the affiliation of the child, but the blood must still be paid for.

Daribi conception theory fits in general with Buckley and Gott-

lieb's stipulation regarding the significance of female blood in reproduction. The Daribi, however, while practicing a very marked separation between the sexes, do not stress greatly the powers of menstrual
blood as such (Wagner 1967, 64 and 1972, 38 ff.; also pers. comm. 1993).
Although it is difficult to develop measures for such a matter cross-culturally, it seems evident to me that, while Daribi and Melpa conception
theory is highly similar, the Melpa stress the dangers of female menstrual blood much more than the Daribi do. Two conclusions result:
one is that ethnotheories must themselves be compared carefully, and
Buckley and Gottlieb's hypothesis is couched too broadly for us to use
it in this context. The second is that, while ideas and beliefs may be similar, different structural or historical conditions may indeed influence
the intensity with which such ideas are inserted into social practices. At
this level, that of practice, variables such as affinal enmity/amity,
which Meggitt, for example, introduced, do become highly relevant. In
other words, both cultural and sociological arguments need to be
advanced, but they must also be hierarchically organized. One set of
factors bears on the ethnobiological theories of the people and the
entailments of these theories in relation to conception. A second set
deals with the expressive significance of such theories within their
structural and pragmatic settings. A failure to distinguish between
these levels of analysis leads investigators to express puzzlement that
theories of conception, for example, are not always isomorphic with
social practices such as rules of descent. If there is isomorphism, it has
to be sought in the relevant domain. Thus, the Daribi and Melpa images
of semen binding or containing (in Melpa *kum ronom* [it makes a pack-
age] female blood introduces an idea of male agency giving form to
female creative substance that is in line with other aspects of male ideology in these societies. Blood may be seen as the bearer of life force
and semen as the power to control or shape this force. But such a stress
on male agency does not necessarily lead to a rigid emphasis on patrilineal descent rules. Blood also may be a basis for affiliation, as the
Daribi example makes abundantly clear.

   The most powerful point made by Buckley and Gottlieb is perhaps
their insistence that an approach via "pollution theory" is only a partial
and one-sided exercise. We can go further and argue that such an
approach in fact accedes to the partial ideologies of males in the cultures we study. Anna Meigs (1984), in her account of the Hua people of
the Eastern Highlands Province, has given a very balanced account of

ideas these people entertain regarding menstruation. She points out that sexual differences are expressed to a great extent by the Hua through food taboos. Generally, foods that are "soft" are considered female, and those that are "hard" or strong are classified as male. Both sexual and alimentary acts are spoken of as transfers of *nu* (juice or life force). Males argue that the transfer of their *nu* as semen increases the female's vitality and decreases that of the male (41). This is a kind of prototypical zero-sum theory that is commonly held by males throughout the Highlands. The Hua have ideas that parallel exactly those of the ancient Greeks: they think that semen originates in the head. They deduce that balding in men is a result of semen loss, a condition they conceal by wearing small woven caps (again, a common practice throughout the Highlands: nowadays men sometimes wear tea cosies instead of such caps, and pushing or detaching a man's cap to show that he is bald is a severe form of insult to his dignity). Females, by contrast, deny that they profit from men's semen, arguing that intercourse actually increases their menstrual flow and thus entails for them also a loss of *nu*. True feeding, however, replenishes *nu* and is considered essentially as a female act. If this is so, it follows that in this regard, at least, females are superior to males. Yet in discussions within their men's houses, away from women, men maintain that their sexual acts "feed" women, while women's acts of feeding can "pollute" them.

In addition, Meigs points out that Hua origin stories (like those of their neighbors and close cultural congeners, the Gimi) suggest a primordial superiority of females (see Gewertz 1988), a theme that is mirrored by the acts of Hua men in imitating menstruation (Meigs cites here also the example of Wogeo men's purification practices described by Hogbin [1970, 88]. Hua men also think that they can become pregnant as a result of a fetus entering the penis (Meigs 1984, 47), an idea they share with their neighbors the Gimi (Glick 1963, 117). The fetus has to be removed by a special operation, since the men obviously cannot give birth to it nor nourish it inside themselves. Hua men also secretly consume foods identified with the "juicy, soft, and cool" qualities of women, to counteract their own "hard, dry, hot" bodies. These facts show that, while the Hua make a sharp distinction between the sexes, this distinction is mediated in a number of ways. Living people in their life cycle also vary in terms of their male and female qualities. We see also the importance of humoral ideas turning on a hot-cold dichotomy, a theme that is found right across the Highlands region from east to west and also in the Madang region among the Yupno people (Keck 1992).

The example of the Hua thus shows clearly that there is a dialectical set of ideas regarding the categories female and male at work, and this corresponds exactly to Buckley and Gottlieb's caveat regarding approaches that simply stress female pollution. Meigs's creative demonstration that for the Hua actual individuals vary in terms of their gendered identity over their life cycle adds a further valuable insight, providing the context in which the dialectic of ideas is played out. The theme of males imitating menstruation is, of course, one that has also attracted the notice of counter-Freudian psychoanalysts such as Bruno Bettelheim ([1954] 1962). In ethnographic terms we can note further that voluntary forms of self-purification by letting blood from *some part* of the body are common in many cultures and were indeed a part of the pre-biomedical European medical tradition based on an idea of balance between humors. Such practices depend on ethnotheories of growth and well-being. In the Hua case men think that, following menstruation, a woman's health improves and that menarche leads to a spurt of growth on the part of the female adolescent (ideas that no doubt have some physiological basis). They let blood from a man's stomach to release supposed clots of blood in him and explain that this would be unnecessary if men could menstruate (Meigs 1984, 56). Hua men also eat plants with a red juice to induce diarrhea and hence purging; Hua women, by contrast, avoid these plants, since consumption of them would cause their menstrual flow to be too heavy (58). We see from this example how characteristics of color and substance can form the basis of symbolic equations. The Hua further explicitly associate the oil of the red pandanus fruit with menstrual blood (32) and forbid its consumption to male initiates. Yet this same food is highly prized in many parts of the Highlands because of its association with blood and strength in general. Melpa men, for example, say that "it helps their blood" to consume it. And Duna men, who have rigid taboos against contact with a menstruating woman, prize red pandanus greatly, insisting only that, if they are to consume it, it must not be squeezed or mixed by a woman.

I give one further example here to show the complications involved in relating ethnotheories to practice. The Gimi, next door to the Hua, hold to a rather unusual conception ideology, that a child is made exclusively from father's semen, not from a mixture of semen and blood. Gimi men argue that their semen "dies" inside the woman and "turns to blood" (Gillison 1993, 210). Conception is seen as a kind of defeat of the Moon, who induces menstruation in women (and whom Gillison equates, via psychoanalytic ideas, with the woman's father). Pregnancy is seen as a complex event, induced both by repeated acts of intercourse with the human husband, imputed intercourse with the Moon, and a dream of seeing ancestral spirits, *kore;* but the woman's own menstrual blood does not contribute to the body of the child.

Nevertheless, menstrual blood is considered in some sense as unclean (the Gimi think that birthing blood is in a sense the "filth of the Moon" and in that sense equate it with menstrual blood). Missionaries in the 1960s did away with the traditional huts for menstrual seclusion, but ideas connected with these persist. A menstruating woman should not walk in the gardens; she should not hold with her hand sweet potatoes she eats but, instead, skewer these with a stick; she discards the tampon of "hot" blood into a deep river; and purifies herself with "blood songs" before resuming the work of cooking for her husband (Gillison 1993, 178). Should she fail to do this, her husband's skin would dry up; he would be pale and fall ill (179). Gimi ideas in this and other spheres are complex, since menstrual blood is held to be a part of the husband (transformed semen). The husband can thus be harmed through ingestion of his own altered substance, cycled through a woman, and "menstrual pollution" in this case is like self-pollution or autocannibalism. Gimi men also let blood from their noses "to rid themselves of accumulations of female blood that dull their skins and sap their strength" (183). The nose is symbolically equated with the penis here, so that Gimi actions closely resemble those of the Wogeo described by Hogbin. One way of referring to menstruation is to say that the Red Lorikeet bird has put his bleeding nose into the woman's vagina (188). Gillison further suggests that menarche represents a first birth from inside the woman, which is a symbolic expulsion of her father (a psychoanalytic way of referring to what the Siane people of the Eastern Highlands celebrate as a birth of paternal spirit on the father's land [Salisbury 1965]). And she concludes that "menstrual blood is both deadly and fertilizing"; it is ambivalent. The woman's blood is also like her own crops and pigs, which for that reason she must not eat (195). All of these facts show the complex articulation of Gimi ideas with practices and indicate again that ethnotheories have themselves to be investigated carefully. The category of "menstrual blood involved in reproduction" is too broad for us to work with it as an explanatory variable in itself. But the Gimi materials abundantly confirm the proposition that menstrual blood may be both dangerous and beneficent, a proposition that undercuts pure sociological approaches based on the idea of "danger" by showing that the cultural dimension does not allow for such an oversimplified view.

Conception Theories and the Life Cycle

Gimi conception theory reveals a triadic pattern: a child is made when (1) there is an accumulation of semen inside a woman, (2) the woman has a particular dream of ancestral spirits (kore), (3) the Moon permits/collaborates in the overall process. The particular constellation of ideas here is rather unusual, but the division between what we might be tempted to call physical and metaphysical factors is typical. It is better, however, not to use our own categories of the physical and the metaphysical here, since all of the factors involved may have both a material and a spiritual aspect. Ideas to do with growth and with giving birth, and subsequently nurture, to the child belong to the same logical set as ideas of conception itself. Women possess the power to make plants and pigs grow by singing songs to them (Gillison 1993, 159), endowing them with agency and flattering them by comparing them to beautiful things of the wild forest areas that grow easily and in profusion. They join their *auna* (spirit) with that of the plants and make them grow well (199), like the *korena*, "wild things."

There is more than metaphor or simile involved in these magical songs. *Auna* is the force that animates a person, and at death it flies out of the fontanelle as a newborn child emerges from the vagina, or as semen emerges at ejaculation, and enters at first "wind, rivers and marsupials, and later entering Birds of Paradise, giant trees, mountain caves and every form of forest life" (200). In this wild environment, which is equated with the world of spirit, production takes place effortlessly. A woman's ability to mimic this power of production is derived from her menstrual blood, but this in turn derives from male semen, so the Gimi have a strongly male-biased theory of the ultimate origins of life force in the world. In addition their theories are strongly cyclical. The *auna* of the dead is ejected into the forest and increases its fertility, so the game that men bring back as food from the forest is impregnated with ancestral force and thus reanimates the living. And conception itself depends on the entry into the head of a sleeping woman by an ancestral *kore* spirit, who thereby gives the woman a dream: if she dreams of a frog, her child will be female; if of a bird, it will be male. This entry into the head is described by the Gimi as a kind of spirit "trick," and Gillison also glosses it as a form of copulation. We see here the fusion of "material and spiritual" that I referred to earlier; or perhaps we see simply a different theory of "material" happenings. In any case, *kore* and *auna* are implicated in conception, death, the return of spirit in food, and thus in growth. No stage of the life cycle is free from the pervasive influence of *kore*.

The omnipresence of *kore* entails precautions on the part of an expectant father also. The man must not enter a *neki maha* forest place, where "moisture-laden plants grow in profusion" (Gillison 1993, 224). He might by chance incur the anger of creatures or plants there that will curse him and steal some of his *auna*, which otherwise he would impart to his child. *Neki maha* places also hold the *auna* of children who died young or were miscarried, and these hold a grudge against the living and so must not be offended. To cool the anger of a spirit a man will try to collect running water and pour it over his sick child's head. He takes this water from the forest place where he had earlier offended the spirit (228). Gillison suggests that the water represents also the man's own substance, which he gives to the child to make it well. "Substance" here is always bound up with *auna* (spirit).

The Gimi case indicates clearly aspects of the person that are connected to their conception theories: a person is always animated by and is dependent on the variable presence of *auna*, whether derived from the actual intrusion of a spirit or the spirit element in food. The forest is the repository of spirit force: life comes from it and returns to it; it is the epitome of the overall cycle. Yet, this generalized force cannot be equated with individual consciousness, or knowledge, will, and intention. *Mind, knowledge,* and *willpower* do not occur in Gillison's index. Semen and *auna* are needed to make the child, but what makes the child fully human?

My model here for raising this question is the Melpa case. Melpa believe that semen binds blood and makes the body of the child, which is further quickened by the action of ancestral spirits in implanting a *min*, so that when the child is born it already shows the presence of *min* by its breathing (A. J. Strathern 1972, 9–10). As Hermann Strauss explains (1990, 99 ff.), the *min* is in some sense separable from the body, appearing as shadow or image and leaving it at death, but when the person is conscious and well the *min* is in every part of the body, so that any bodily emission entails a loss of *min* also. *Min* is clearly similar to *auna,* or the Hua *aune,* as well as to a range of concepts cited by Meigs (1984, 129) from other New Guinea cultures. For the Melpa *min* is especially associated with the hair and the head as a whole. But the child when born does not have a *noman,* or "mind." This develops only over time, as the child learns to speak (A. J. Strathern 1980, 1994) and as it develops an awareness of social relations and its own volitional choices. It is especially interesting to me to see whether this Melpa concept of *noman* is paralleled in other Highlands cultures, yet it is also in this regard that evidence is hardest to find. "Mind" has not been a problem of concern to either Gillison or Meigs in their studies of the Gimi and Hua, and it is therefore hard to complete one's picture of the person and personhood for these people, in spite of the rich ethnographic data on the body, on menstruation, and on conception. Yet the minds of kinsfolk are clearly at work among the Gimi: mother's brothers may utter curses and cause sickness, for example. Perhaps the "vehicle" involved is always *auna,* but some concept of mind as cause may perhaps also be present.

In conception theories themselves this mindful element is represented both in the implicit intentionality of the parents in having sex (described by the Melpa as "work" *[kongon]*) and also in the activities of spirit agencies who will or oversee the subsequent conception and birth. The image of intentionality or agency may also bridge over into male ideology, when it is asserted, for example as among the Gimi, that a child is formed only from the father's semen and further that menstrual blood itself is transformed semen. Barth reports for the Baktaman that a child is held to spring entirely from the father's semen. Mother's blood nourishes it, hence the cessation of menstruation, but does not give it essential substance, which is shared only by the father and his clan (Barth 1975, 77). (The exclusiveness of this ideology appears to be negated, however, by Mackenzie's data [see Mackenzie 1991].) If we now look at a small number of cases in some further detail, we may be able to pinpoint the variable place of ideology and intentionality more closely.

I take first the Paiela, whose ideas have been outlined earlier. Biersack argues that for these people *no* magicoreligious beliefs as such are at work in relation to conception. Her starting point derives from an earlier, and rather misconceived, debate about the idea of "virgin birth" among the Trobrianders (see also Delaney 1986). The Trobrianders stress the cosmic role of *baloma* clan spirits in conception and thereby in a sense downplay the physical role of *both* parents in the process (although mother's blood is held to form the child's bodily substance). In particular, at least traditionally and within dogmatic contexts, they deny that semen has a procreative role to play, although they allow that the husband's intercourse with his wife molds the child in his wife's womb, an idea whose effect is not unlike that of the Daribi view that semen forms the outer part of a child's body. Biersack takes up the cosmological side of the equation. If Trobrianders overstress it, Paiela understress it, at least in surface terms. "Spirits" are apparently not involved. We might enter here a caveat. The Paiela physical doctrine is closely similar to that of the Melpa. Melpa also consider, however, that a child's *min* is derived from ancestral agency, and furthermore they hold (as do the Gimi) that the dead father of a woman may prevent her from producing a child if the father died angry over an exchange debt or a refusal to give him pork or to care for him in old age (A. J. Strathern 1993b, 7). In the Melpa case causation lies with the will, or mind, of the spirits: physical processes do not take place automatically or autonomously. Spirits are invoked to account for infertility and to attempt its redress through sacrifices of pigs.

Biersack's purpose is to assign conception theories to their correct local domain of discourse, and she argues that the Paiela theory in fact relates to social structure rather than to procreation. Here she alters the terms of previous discussions considerably. Discussions tend to focus on the interrelationship *between* conception theories and social structure, whereas Biersack argues that these *are* theories about social structure. She refers to them also as acts of "metaphorical modelling" (1983, 93). In Paiela marriage practices a major aim is to transform unrelated (unbound) groups to intermarrying ones, and intermarriage is therefore a kind of "binding," an act of joining across a boundary. Conception theory thus models the social act of intermarrying. If this is so, however, another element is also involved: gender hierarchy. As she explains, the male is represented as active in the sexual transaction, since it is he who pays bridewealth and approaches the woman for intercourse. Thus, it is semen that binds blood. (Agency, as we have earlier seen, is described as *nembo*, mind or choice-making capacity, which is also seen as surviving death, although there is no theory of its recycling into newborn children.) This element of gender hierarchy, reflecting male agency, links the Paiela to the Melpa and Daribi cases, even though the organization of sexual reproduction is not exactly the same in all three cases. But why should we argue, or conclude, from these observations that conception theory is not, after all, about procreation but *only* about social structure, appealing to the idea of metaphor as the bridge between these two? It would be more parsimonious to argue that a conception theory is itself an element in a wider theory of gender relations that organizes many domains of social life. Such an argument avoids the difficulties of a "reflectionist" position that the body "symbolizes" society, as also the claim that a conception theory is actually not about conception but about structure. The operation of thought here is metonymous rather than metaphorical: conception theory is indeed a part of a theory of cosmic and social structure, a theory that privileges male agency and mind as a moving force. Yet we have also seen that this hierarchical notion is itself reversed in the image of the ginger-woman, who rules over the growth of boys just as the married man putatively "rules" over his wife by binding her menstrual blood with his semen.

In Biersack's analysis it is male ideology that is in focus. Jorgensen, writing on the Telefolmin, provides a case in which men and women have different versions of ideas about conception (Jorgensen 1983). The Telefolmin belong to the Ok region west of Paiela. Like the Paiela they have named cognatic categories *(tenum miit)* but these do not produce corporate groupings. Gender, however, does provide a basic structural dimension (58), one that therefore also encompasses the investigator.

Telefolmin men were reluctant, not to say embarrassed, to discuss conception and childbirth with Jorgensen. They declared that the topic was awkward enough to put men off eating and agreed finally to produce a statement only because it was Jorgensen's "work" to acquire information on the topic. They consistently told him he should really ask the women about this. What they eventually told him was much in line with statements made by men in neighboring cultures—in the case of the Duna also with some reluctance—but with at least one difference. They declared that babies were formed, from "penis water" and "vaginal fluid." Several acts of intercourse were needed to build up the fetus, but after the fetus was there intercourse should cease; otherwise, twins would form. As Jorgensen notes, this "symmetrical" notion of conception fits, in a mild fashion, with the cognatic quality of Telefol kinship (Jorgensen 1983, 59). More specific ties are built up with parents *after* birth through nurturance and care. Indeed, the idea that semen "feeds" the child in the womb is one that is found elsewhere in Melanesia, so nurturing can begin even before birth. In the Telefol men's version, however, one element is missing: blood. In the women's account this was brought in and made central. They agreed that a child is initially formed by sexual fluids but added that menstrual blood makes the child's *bones*. These same bones become the focus, after the person's death, of male ritual activity designed to restimulate powers of growth in the cosmos, and from this activity women are firmly excluded. By the women's version, therefore, "the chief relics of the men's cult (bones) find their source in the very substance (menstrual blood) which the men find abhorrent" (61). We have already seen a similar paradox with regard to the *bagan isak* paint used to decorate initiates. *Isak* in fact means "blood," and the provenance of the paint has entirely to do with female blood, although it is also associated with male ancestors. We are dealing here with an interesting crossover of ideas. Men's use of menstrual blood as an ingredient in paint indicates a covert "knowledge" of its positive powers (not, incidentally, communicated to the initiates themselves). They profess, however, not to know what such blood contributes to in conception (creating, as Jorgensen notes, a "deafening silence" on the matter). Either we are dealing again with a covert recognition or with a unilateral claim by the women that their power to make bones, seen as white, from red blood is celebrated in the men's cult. In any case, the men's and women's versions have to be seen as "in a dialectical relationship," in which the women's account represents a secret "increment" to the men's, a "marked" as against the "unmarked" version that both sexes share.

Jorgensen further notes that red-white transformations occur in other cultic contexts also. The men's cult congregation is divided into two halves, one associated with nurturance, taro growing, and the color white; the other with killing, warfare and hunting, and the color red. Nurturance and killing are held to be antithetical yet complementary, and on occasion they are brought into ritual concordance. Thus, at the time of the taro harvest a pig is slaughtered in the garden, and its blood must flow into the ground: red assists in "giving birth" to white. The process here can be seen as analogous to that whereby menstrual blood (red) creates bone (white). Jorgensen gives a set of further examples, two belonging to the opposite point in the life cycle from conception: death. (1) At death a corpse is placed on an exposure platform; its flesh and blood fall into the ground (contributing to fertility?), and the white bones are gathered for cult use. (2) In a secret myth, cowrie valuables (white) used as "vital wealth" in life cycle payments emerge "from maggots in the rotting flesh of a corpse" (Jorgensen 1983, 62). If we see the flesh as red, this is another case of white produced from red. Red is powerful, if ambivalent; white is a "result," a purified "state" resting on a prior process of creation.

These two examples raise other issues. One is the place of the body in the total cycle of cosmic reproduction. A second is the theme of the human body as the source of crops or valuables, the body as the creator of fertility and wealth. Both themes are taken up further in later pages.

Thus far we have discussed Telefolmin theories of conception, the body, and ritual power in "substance" terms. But there is a further Telefolmin concept, *sinik*, which "comprises the notion of awareness and personality as well as the physiognomy that distinguishes one individual from another" (Jorgensen 1983, 59). *Sinik* implies the ability to hear and understand others and is signaled by the child's acquisition of speech (exactly as the Melpa say *noman* is attained). It therefore grows as the child grows and is not implanted during conception. How does *sinik* interact with substance? Clues to this problem can be found in Mackenzie's work and perhaps also in Poole's writings on the Bimin-Kuskusmin, who live to the southeast of Telefomin. Mackenzie discusses the making of a sacred *iman men* net bag belonging to the Taro moiety, within which the bones of a corpse will be housed. (She notes that in the case of a female corpse the mouth is filled with *red ocher,* representing the creatrix Afek's menstrual blood.) "The taro side expert then addresses the *sinik* (spirit) of the corpse, telling it that the villagers would like it to remain with them to be an *using* (ancestor spirit) and not turn into a *bagel* (ghost spirit) and go to Bagelam (the Land of the Dead)" (Mackenzie 1991, 123). After the corpse decays, the expert collects certain bones (skull, forearm, finger, wrist, ankle) and places them in the string bag, where the ancestor spirit can be "reborn" "within the womb-like sanctuary" (123). Each village needs its spirit string bags and bones as a means to its power and well-being, but the bags have to be well attended, for they could also be dangerous, particularly to women. Red cordyline bushes are planted as taboo signs in front of the men's house where these bones are kept, since these bushes are also repositories of *sinik* and will whistle warnings to the *using* on the approach of trespassers. *Using* are considered to be sentient and individual: they hear prayers and rattle their bones in reply, and they like their bones to be rubbed with pig fat. If neglected, they refuse to help their curators (182–83). It is plain that *sinik* and *using* represent the extension of individual identity and mind into the period after death. The bones that hold this identity are like its "house," just as cult stones are described by Duna male informants as the "house" of spirits.

Telefolmin men could apparently not account for the first development of *sinik* and did not see it as transmitted or recycled through conception. The Bimin have a closely related concept, *finiik*, which enters into a complex system of gender ideas based on procreation and the life cycle. While I cannot deal here with the full articulation of these ideas, it is useful to note that they all seem to be substance based, in the sense that they posit the transmission of capacities via conception and the ingestion of food. *Finiik* is primarily a male procreative contribution, which has to be strengthened by infusions of male blood or semen at times of crisis, breast milk (seen as derived from the mother's own male-transmitted fluids), and male foods (e.g., pandanus nuts, taro, pork, marsupial meat), and by ritual activities (Poole 1985, 198). As the person grows up, *finiik* comes to have the meanings of will, desire, intention, consciousness, understanding, motivation, concentration, and social competence (exactly the range of the Melpa *noman*): in summary it becomes "the ordered, controlled, careful, thoughtful, socially proper aspects of personality and self." At the beginning of life, however, it is already imparted by "an undifferentiated corpus of ancestral spirits" who guide its development. In death "it departs from the body to enter the corpus of ancestral spirits from which it originated and to return to the living in the form of a new baby, of its own volition or when summoned by ritual activity" (199).

Finiik carries male gender associations and is strengthened by male substances and actions. A different kind of spirit, *khaapkabuurien* is supposed to be derived from vapors in the mother's womb linked to her own emotions. It is capricious and entirely the product of individual experience and it balances against the *finiik*. At death it may become a wandering and dangerous ghost unless it is integrated with the *finiik* to become an ancestral spirit. In this dual conception of the soul, or spirit, the Bimin show a stress on gender hierarchy, comparable to the Paiela, and also tie this to an implicitly agnatic ideology, an element that appears to differentiate them from the Telefolmin. Their ideas are a permutation of ones shared by others in their region: *finik* is also reported by Barth on the Baktaman as the "spirit, soul, or consciousness" that survives death (Barth 1975, 124).

Generalizing from these cases, we can suggest that the element of mind may be seen as intersecting with body in a number of different ways: (1) it may be equated with life force and be seen as recycled into and out of bodies with the help of ancestral agency (Gimi); (2) it may be seen as transmitted or acquired in a variety of ways, some substance based and others not, and aspects of it seen as recycled over the generations (Bimin); (3) it may be conceptualized as a separate dimension of the person, intimately linked with the body and dying with it, in contrast to a transmitted or recycled soul (Melpa), or as itself turning into the soul (Paiela, Telefolmin). These different conjunctures further have different implications for the sickness and health of the person, a theme I explore in the next chapter.

Another feature of the data I have been discussing is the parallelism between birth and death, which is most apt to be stressed in the context of an overall theory of cyclicity. For the Gimi, the release of the *auna* from the dead body is explicitly seen as a kind of birth (or a procreative act of "ejaculation," as Gillison puts it). And Mackenzie points out that for the Telefolmin a sacred net bag containing selected bones of a dead person is the "womb" inside which a new ancestral spirit comes into being. These two conceptualizations also differ in their implications. The Gimi *auna* recycles into the forest, contributing there to generalized fertility and power, while the Telefolmin *sinik* "reconceives" itself as an individual agent of power on behalf of a particular set of people and thus able to influence the individual bodies of its living kin, as does the Melpa *min* or soul when it turns at death into a *kor* (although for the Melpa the person's *noman* as such does not survive death).

Skin and Its Capacities

Roy Wagner, in the course of his essay on conception ideas among the Daribi and the Barok of New Ireland (1983), tells us something about Daribi ideas of skin and the body system, ideas that mesh with those on conception itself. According to accounts given by Daribi women, and relayed to their men on Wagner's behalf, "the human body contains two networks of tubes: the outer, or *agwa* system, which we call the lymphatic system, and which is said to contain semen in men (in women it contributes to maternal milk) and the inner or blood system, with its veins and arteries" (76). Women always have enough blood inside them, but men have strictly limited quantities of semen and must augment their supply of this substance through eating meat, which they share with paternal kinsmen. The self-sufficient power of fertility in women has also to be paid off by prestations of male-controlled wealth: there is a flow of wealth against fertility, as there is a flow of semen into women themselves. In both cases contingent male resources are mobilized in order to encompass self-sufficient female resources.

The ideas that semen (related to fat, juice, or water) is located in a system of "veins" throughout the body just underneath the surface of the skin and that it is in finite supply are not peculiar to the Daribi. Whether it is articulated so precisely as by the Daribi women (and it is notable that they were the ones openly to draw attention to the matter) or not, there is a widespread perception on the part of men in a range of Melanesian cultures that their potential to produce semen is limited and that shortage of it results in skin that is dry, loose, or discolored and flaky, as though it had ashes on it. It is exactly this condition of men's skin, as noted earlier, that is also held to result from inappropriate contact with menstrual blood. Sexual intercourse is thus seen as inexorably sapping men's vital juices, making them old, and intercourse with a menstruating woman is bound to accelerate this lethal process further, because the blood of menstruation itself is thought of in this context as "dry" and dead.

The condition of a man's skin is therefore a direct reflection of his current sexual situation. The Melpa are not so forthcoming as are the Daribi about the need for men to consume pork in order to maintain their semen levels, but they are very clear that a "bad" skin is a result of overindulgence in sex or exposure to pollution. Skin therefore is not just a sign of vitality but an index also of one's personal and moral state. The Melpa go further and argue that all conditions of the "body"—that is, the skin or outer visible part of the person—are a result of the inner condition of the *noman*, or mind. If persons looks well and their skin is big, they are asked first what kind of *noman* they currently have. Obviously, it must be a good state of the *noman*, they reason, because this is evinced by the good state of the skin.

This same theory of the skin is found among the Paiela. We have seen how they think of fat or juice as growing in the inner skin and how their bachelors ask for the ginger-woman's help in producing this fat by her coming and "sitting in their skin." Skin is therefore the sign of the choice of this female spirit to help the youths to become "big" and "beautiful." The ginger-woman's presence within their inner skin makes their outer skin attractive. We see here a paradigm of inner skin as cause and outer skin as effect, analogous to the Melpa image of the (inner) *noman* as cause, whose effects also show on the (outer) skin.

The skin is also, from another perspective, the marker of experience, knowledge, and morality. Poole quotes a Bimin text referring to infants who do not yet have a clearly defined basis for personhood: "[the infant] has no "skin" (*kaar*) of its own [i.e., no experience of life, no "shame" (*fiitom*)]" (1985, 183). The Bimin concept that Poole translates as self is literally "skin root" (*kaar kiim kiim*) (185). "Self-centeredness" apparently also has to do with the skin, since the term for it is *kaar dugaamkhaa* (199). It is especially associated with infants, and linked to the weakness among them of *finiik* and the strength of the capricious *khaapkhabuurien* spirit. The term for *hot* is apparently a reduplication of that for skin (*kaar kaar*), suggesting that certain impulses are experienced as heat on the skin (213; my interpretation). The child begins as an amalgam of desire, envy and frustration, all linked to female-derived internal organs such as the gallbladder and spleen, and only gradually learns embarrassment, described as *kaar-kuureng-mamin*, a term that clearly includes again the word for "skin." Later again it learns "shame" (*fiitom*). Embarrassment signals "an infantile recognition of wrongdoing or impropriety that involved both the self and others in relationship" (215). The Bimin concept of skin thus seems to work as the Melpa concept does, making skin the marker of the boundary, and also the connection, between the self and those to whom it is related. This was the answer I gave to the question regarding the Melpa: "Why is shame on the skin?" (A. J. Strathern 1975). Poole in fact provides an elaboration of this point when he writes for the Bimin that "the external, behavioral aspects of shame are "on" (*aar-ker*) the skin and the internal aspects that connote "feeling/thinking badly" are "beneath" (*afaak-ker*) the skin. . . . It is this latter sense that is significantly bound up with the . . . notion of self or skin-root" (Poole 1985, 218). The reference to "beneath the skin" implies a link to the *finiik*, and it is this link therefore that is the "root" that connects the skin to the *finiik*, explaining why it can be affected by the *finiik*. Self thus appears to be the connection between outer "appearance" and inner "consciousness," all expressed in bodily terms.

The Bimin also subscribe to the idea that a gendered array of foods must be consumed to assist in the development of the gendered person. In many Highlands cultures such consumption extends even to contexts of initiation, which frequently involve the expulsion of female or maternal blood in males and the ingestion or consumption of "male foods," in some cases semen itself (as, e.g., among the Sambia or Simbari Anga and the Etoro [Herdt 1982; Kelly 1977]). Whether we argue that this reflects a transformation from an initially androgynous to a single-gendered state depends on the way the term *androgynous* is taken. Most specifically, the ideas involved have to do with "weakening" and "strengthening" influences, seen as the effect of gendered substances, and we might prefer to argue that it is these substances that are applied as an increment that can make a difference in the body of an initially "sexed" but not "gendered" initiate. Such an argument would make it unnecessary to invoke *androgyny*, a term with a physiological ring to it, although Bimin culture at least does contain certain images of androgyny with respect to the creative ancestress Afek and her brother Yomnok.

What is clearly evident is that the Bimin men consider that male substances and foods are needed to make boys male. A father transfuses his blood into his infant son when the boy is given a "female name" at roughly two years of age (Poole 1985, 194). He may feed mashed taro coated with human or boar semen to an unweaned infant who is seriously ill (231). At the time of full initiation female blood and breast milk are ritually driven out of the boys, and they are required to ingest male foods: "ground-dwelling bird eggs, river moss, red mushrooms, toads, and land crabs," accompanied always by taro and ginger (Poole 1982, 124, 132).

This gendered logic of consumption is also found very markedly among the Hua. Vital fluid in the body, *nu*, has to be maintained in balance. "The male, having a relatively small amount of *nu*, has difficulty in growing in his adolescent years and in maintaining adequate vitality in his adult years. The female, because of her inherently greater endowment of *nu*, grows fast, ages slowly, and maintains her vitality" (Meigs 1984, 27). Males are at risk of having too little, females of having too much, *nu*, in fact. Adolescent male initiates are accordingly required to eat food that are *korogo*, "juicy," to help them grow (the concern here is the same as that among the Paiela) whereas a menstruating woman should eat substances that are *hakeri'a*, "hard and slow-growing," in order to return her body to a more dry state. The *nu* in menstrual blood can also be dangerous to initiates, who should therefore avoid red foods that are associated with this substance (28) as well as abstain from a whole further set of items that are reminiscent of female parts. Several foods carry a sexual connotation, and Meigs recognizes a general parallelism between the "sexual and alimentary systems" (36), with a special equation between the vagina and the mouth. *Nu* is transferred in all acts of eating and in all bodily emissions, and all such acts conduce to growth or decline of the body. Sexual intercourse depletes a man's *nu* and accelerates his balding, since semen is believed to originate in the head. Women deny that they gain men's *nu*, however, and stress that they themselves lose too much *nu* in menstruation. Each sex is therefore greatly concerned about achieving the correct balance of *nu* within the body, and each attempts to adjust this balance through consumption of "gendered" foods. Meigs describes this process, with its linked moral values, as a "physical metaphor" (40), but it is doubtful if the Hua see this as a metaphor at all. For them it is a straightforward set of acts that have, for them, a biological value and amount to an "ideology of life" (29).

Both males and females also attempt positively to influence the balance of *nu* within themselves, as we have seen. As Meigs notes, "for the female to reproduce, she must be extremely *korogo* [soft, wet]; for the male to defend himself and her, he must be extremely *hakeri'a* [hard, dry]" (1984, 88). Indeed, this aim of manipulating the body's essences forms a major part of Hua religion, such that Meigs appropriately entitles the final chapter of her book "A Religion of the Body." Finally, she emphasizes that for the Hua female *nu* is the most plentiful and powerful, so that, when men wish to augment their own *nu*, one way in which they do this is by imitation of female powers and ingestion of female-linked substances. Thus, "in this religion of the body the female body plays the star role" (131).

The Hua do not appear to have greatly elaborated the role of the skin in social communication regarding the body. They stress rather the imputed internal state of the body, achieved through observance of eating rules. Another people in the Eastern Highlands of Papua New Guinea do emphasize the skin, however, and their ideas to do with it have formed the basis of a further argument about individuality and the concept of the person. These are the Gahuku-Gama, described by Read (1955).

Read's argument was that for the Gahuku-Gama there was "no essential separation of the individual from the social pattern: social roles and social status are not distinguished from the individuals who enact them" (Read 1955, 276; qtd. in LaFontaine 1985, 129). He contrasted Gahuku ideas further with Christian ones, arguing that in the former there is no generalized concept of a person (human being) that could be made the basis of a universal or extended morality. Langness (1987, 19) quickly notes that Christian practice may be different from theory and also that the absence of a universalizing rule does not mean necessarily the absence of a sentiment of such a universalizing kind. These formulations by Read are peculiarly close, in fact, to ethnocentric glosses based on a civilized-primitive dichotomy. The "primitives" are depicted as having no "real concept" of the individual separate from social roles and, correlatively, no morally universal idea of the person that could transcend their particular society. Elaborate comment on the ethnocentric basis or bias of this picture seems almost unnecessary, but further scrutiny of Gahuku ideas on skin is in order, since this was the focus of Read's own interpretation. Skin and morality are connected, as we have seen them to be among the Melpa and Paiela, for example, and it is this physically embodied imagery that Read took to be diagnostic of a lack of distinction between individual and social role. Debt is said to be "in the skin" (as it is in Melpa). Good or bad skin is a sign of a morally good or bad state.

But what has this to do with the presence or absence of a concept of the individual or the person? LaFontaine defined *individual*, following Fortes, as a "moral human being," and the Gahuku define a part of such morality in terms of the condition of the skin in the body. Still seeking a we-they dichotomy, LaFontaine suggests that the Gahuku "do not distinguish clearly the material and immaterial (including the social) attributes of persons (LaFontaine 1985, 130). This implies that there is some prior, universal, true distinction along these lines. Yet, as she herself notes, there are dangers of ethnocentrism in the discussion. Why should there be such a distinction? It may be in fact that a distinction of this sort is fostered most in societies with "abstract" bureaucracies and legal systems. For the Gahuku, with their embodied, face-to-face social relationships based on direct communication, making the skin one site of morality amounts to good "symbolic sense," and it does not preclude a concept of individual agency or choice, since it is precisely choice that leads to a good or bad condition of the skin, whether this is one's own choice or that of another who feels favorably or disfavorably toward one. Reformulating Read's proposition only to reject it as a solution to a nonexistent dichotomy, LaFontaine suggests that the bodily concepts of the Gahuku "should perhaps be seen as the conceptual mechanism whereby these people obliterate the distinction between an individual and his social roles by incorporating the latter into his physical self, the skin" (130). She rejects this reformulation on the grounds that the Gahuku do not distinguish between actor and role in the first place so they have no need to obliterate this distinction.

My argument, however, is that the distinction between actor and role *is* present and is not obliterated but is actually expressed through the skin idiom. I thus turn both LaFontaine's and Read's arguments inside out. Reading back from "our" folk concepts, they find these missing among the Gahuku and are left with a puzzling (to them) idiom of *the skin*. I am suggesting, however, that, if we "read the skin" (to use a phrase invented by O'Hanlon [1989]) correctly, we can see that it does precisely index the articulation of the inner self (and thus the individual in that sense) with outer social relationships. Misprision of Gahuku ideas on the body thus leads to a misprision of their ideas of morality and the person. Read's own interpretation led him to argue that the Gahuku have no concept of "friendship" (although they did in fact exercise preference in relationships). Here he defined friendship in "Western European" terms as a relationship between two unique individuals not otherwise related. Such a definition is itself somewhat ideological: most actual friendships *are* predicated on social bases and are added to these in a process that is exactly comparable to what occurs among the Gahuku. And, if Gahuku have an idea of friendship based on exchanges of wealth, it is tendentious to argue that this does not qualify as friendship "proper." *Friendship* is a local and ethnographic, not a universal, term.

Another part of Read's argument was that for the Gahuku the *meni,* or life force, does not survive death, even though in life it is "the whole self or personality" (Read 1955, 265; qtd. in LaFontaine 1985, 129). Perhaps we can understand Gahuku concepts better as examples of "cycling" theory such as the Gimi have: if the *meni* contributes to the fertility of the wild at death and returns by multiple pathways to individuals in life, we can see it as a part of a cosmic "humoral" theory, such as the Hua have explicitly articulated in their idea of *nu* (related to the Gimi *auna*). Again, this does not mean that in life there is no concept of the individual: it does mean that this concept is less stressed after death than it is, for example, by the Telefolmin people with their theory of how the *sinik* becomes a *using*, spirit.

If we pursue the theme of the skin and its significance further, we can see how it is used in folktales and in cosmological accounts. The Gimi consider that when persons die their skin is changed: the dark outer skin is removed, and the white inner skin is revealed. This white skin is seen as similar to that of a newborn child. After the Australians entered their area in the 1930s, the Gimi began to "recognize" them as the returned spirits of their own dead (later in this chapter I describe the similar ideas of the Kaliai). Correlatively, they now consider that their own *auna* after death go not to the forest, as in their original cosmology, but down to Australia. Australia has been included in the overall cyclicity of persons, fertility, and wealth, and this inclusion gives the Gimi an unrequited claim, in their own eyes, on Australian goods and wealth and a basis for criticizing white outsiders who do not "share" adequately with them (a common theme in Melanesian history, central to the so-called cargo cult phenomena [see Lindstrom 1993]). My point here is less to comment on the "cargoistic" import of this reshaping of Gimi cosmology, and more to highlight again the significance of the outer-inner opposition. A change of skin is a revelation of inner identity, a turning outside of that which was concealed. Putting it in another way, we can say it is a demonstration of desire, corresponding also to a Lacanian sense of lack.

In folktales this same theme occurs in a widespread set of stories about persons who take off and put on new skins. The underlying image may be that of the snake, which sloughs off its skin and appears young again. As the Melpa and many other peoples say, "we people cannot do that, and so we have to die (*tin wamb tikil ri nö ruimin*, we people will not peel off our skins [and live again])." Folktales and cosmology may deny this "fact" and so "invent immortality" in various ways, one way being perhaps the Gimi assertion that people indeed do take off their skins at death and thereby achieve a new "life" that is in a sense a reversal of their previous one. Folktales portray the same desire in contexts of human interaction that involve reversals and dramatic recognitions between people and that mimic also the dramatized transitions of puberty rites centering on beauty practiced by the Paiela and their neighbors the Duna (Stürzenhofecker 1993) and the Huli (Frankel 1986).

The theme is found already in the work of Malinowski on the Trobrianders, in which he records that the culture hero Kasabwaybwayreta set out in his canoe from Tewara for Wawela in order to obtain a notable spondylus necklace *(soulava)*. On arrival his sons offered betel-nuts, bananas, and coconuts to the hosts, but these were refused until Kasabwaybwayreta spoke magic over them and made them ripe and full and thus acceptable as solicitory gifts *(pokala)*. He then removed his gray hair and his wrinkled skin and left these behind in the canoe. A beautiful man now, he proceeds to charm his host, who agrees to give him the fine necklace, Gumakarakedakeda, which he puts in his hair. Returning to the canoe he resumes his old hair and skin, and his sons are amazed and jealous when they see that he has the valuable necklace—how could an old, ugly man have won this object, which is clearly seen as similar to a woman who has been charmed and given away as a bride by her father? (Malinowski [1922], 1979, 360).

The "inner skin" of Kasabwaybwayreta, representing his desire for the valuable necklace, is "beautiful." Yet, once he has the necklace, he puts his old skin back on again, as apparently he must. He is a dual entity, a combination of opposites, ugly to beautiful, old to young. Skin transformations always involve such reversals. In a Kewa story from Erave in the Southern Highlands of Papua New Guinea, a mother-in-law tricks her new, young daughter-in-law into drowning in a lake and then switches her own old skin with the young skin of the corpse. She impersonates her own daughter-in-law and cooks food for her son as if he were her husband. The little brother of the dead girl reveals what the older woman has done, however, and the son takes revenge on his own mother by killing her and burning her remains in a fire. At night they try to entice the drowned girl back by singing and dancing in a house built over the lake. She comes but shakes the house and departs, making a noise like thunder. The story is given a last-line etiological twist with: "and so this was the origin of thunder" (MacDonald 1991, 370).

In another story from the same area an old couple have a son whose skin is disfigured with scabies. The boy is disobedient, and they plan to kill and cook him. The boy attempts to avoid this fate by stealing his mother's skin and putting it on himself as a disguise (MacDonald 1991, 279). And in a third story there is a young woman called Nugini who has a skin covered in sores. In spite of this, there is a good young man who wishes to marry her. One day the man goes to a dance, and the woman removes her bad skin and hides it beneath her sleeping mat then decorates her (inner) skin (which is good) and visits the dance ground, where she is admired and desired by all the men. She runs home and pulls on her ugly skin. When her man comes back he speaks to her of the girl stranger who attended the dance, and she encourages him to go again the next day. He does so but hides by the pathway to watch. Seeing the beautiful girl go past, he quietly returns to the house, finds the bad skin, and burns it in the fire. The girl returns and demands to have her old skin back, and when denied this she runs away, falls into a hole, and becomes a taro plant (497).

This story contains an element that is paralleled by a whole range of stories from the Sepik region, epitomized in Bernard Narakobi's play *Death of a Muruk* (1982). A man spies on women bathing. He sees that they have removed their cassowary skins prior to washing, and he hides the skin of one young woman, whom he desires, so that she cannot turn back into a cassowary. They marry and have children. One day he insults her, implying that she is not a "real woman." She finds the old cassowary skin where he has hidden it, puts it on, and runs away back into the forest. This Sepik story is in turn paralleled by a cycle of Duna folktales in which a woman (implicitly an incarnation of a female spirit, the Payeme Ima) is captured by a man after turning into a range of trees and wild creatures. They marry and have children, but after a while the man fails to give her meat at a pig kill and abuses her as a "wild creature" when she complains. In revenge she takes her children to the high forest (her realm as a spirit), and, when the husband vainly pursues her there, she turns into a wild pandanus tree and transforms her children into flying foxes or pandanus fruits. The husband, in despair, turns into a fruit dove, a bird with a mournful cooing sound.

It is apparent that these stories form a dense commentary on gender relations, based on a narrative of desire, reciprocity, and revenge. The theme of skin changing belongs to this overall narrative, representing the element of desire, as I have argued: either the desire of the one who changes the skin or the desire of a beholder. In the majority of cases the skin changer is female, and the context of transformation is sexual. The same holds for those stories of transformation lacking the skin change motif. When a return to the old state, however, is denied or if the skin changer is insulted, she may take revenge by escaping and/or turning into another object. Her wild, regenerative power is shown by her ability to turn into a fruit or nut tree or a valued crop such as taro.

LeRoy, in his study of Kewa narratives, has devoted a chapter to exploring the theme of skin changers (1985, 180–97). His account suggests that it is not by chance that skin change stories reflect crucial transformations from wild to domestic, old to young, which serve also as commentaries on mortality and the transition between life and death. As I have already noted, in many mythologies the snake is the prototype of the immortal creature because it sheds its skin. The Kewa add to this image symbols of a kind of tree *(pipi)* that sheds its bark and the caddis fly *(yakura),* which sheds its skin, or pupa, and emerges in its final form. Men's ability to renew themselves in this way was putatively lost when a Wiru man from Pangia came and said the Kewa should say "dying, growing up" instead of *"pipi-e, yakura-e"* (181).

Skin changing evokes liminality between statuses and the desire for change that underlies such liminality. From another viewpoint it reflects that distinction between the individual (or the self) and role that Read denied to the Gahuku-Gama. LeRoy is able to show for the Kewa that one set of skin changing stories is modeled on the image of the poor man (paralleled by "ghost" or "enemy"), seen as the peripheral person who threatens a central hierarchy of male power and influence. In my terms the poor man desires to reverse his social condition (equated with his outer skin) and therefore seeks to alter this skin itself. He does not draw on a new skin but merely reveals his true, inner skin as good and beautiful. The Kewa are a society with big men as leaders: prominent entrepreneurs who make their careers by achieving status in exchanges of wealth. In this kind of society the big man is conventionally associated with having a good skin, with plenty of "grease" in it, while the poor man's skin is dry and as though covered with ashes (thus also like a skin defiled by menstrual blood). The Melpa state this explicitly; a rubbish man is *wuö korpa kik,* "a poor ashes man."

The narrative that LeRoy gives in this context is basically the same as that of the girl Nugini cited already but with a poor man as the central skin changer. A young woman insults a poor man who has a miraculous ability to walk on water and transport people safely across a river. Nevertheless, she goes to his house and sees he has much pork there, which he says he is just "looking after" for its owner. She visits a dance and sees there a handsome young man called Ipakeala who has earlier betrothed her. She eventually guesses that this is none other than the poor man in whose house she is staying, and she secretly finds and destroys his old, wrinkled, ashy skin then confronts Ipakeala with having deceived her. He replies that he did so only in annoyance at her original insults to him in his guise as a poor man and that now she must never refer to his past. She bears him a son, but one day they quarrel about who should clean up the child's feces (which are considered to pollute the skin and make it look old). The woman tells him that he is not a big man, only a poor man, so he can clean the feces from the floor. In anger the man takes his son into the forest, where they turn into tree ferns (wild, decorative, not fertile). The wife sings a mourning lament and turns into a Job's tears plant (worn as a sign of mourning by Kewa women).

The story combines two sequences of recognitions and reversals, centered not on a woman, as in the other Kewa version and in Duna stories, but on a poor man. LeRoy gives further stories, however, that do make a woman or girl the chief skin changer and identifies the basic semantic contrasts as between (1) home and dancing ground (2) ashes and wealth, and (3) death and life. Ashes mark poverty, but they *also* are invoked in spells to effect transformation. LeRoy suggests "they mediate between the domestic and the ceremonial, perhaps because of the transformative capacities of fire and cooking" (1985, 189). As he also notes (297), they mark liminality and in this respect play a similar role among the Kewa to that found in Cinderella and Assipattle stories in European folktales (Grierson 1938).

In another formulation LeRoy suggests that the stories disclose the opposition between "flamboyant ceremony and routine home life," a "social duality" that the skin changer (male) exemplifies "by means of his individual duality" (LeRoy 1985, 191). In the case of females the contrast is between immature girls and grown females, whereas for males it is between old, senile men and handsome youths. Summarizing, he argues that in domestic space "the male realizes himself as old or impoverished, and the female realizes herself as ungrown, unattractive and inadequate. In a ceremonial space, on the other hand, both are alive and vital, physically and spiritually enhanced" (192). Most generally, "an outer change stands for an inner transformation; two skins stand for two roles," and, finally, "the body is a metaphor for the spirit within" (197).

LeRoy"s conclusions are insightful. Accepting them, I wish only to place them in a slightly different perspective, to rephrase them. The drive of his analysis is to display the social categories involved and the representation of their duality within the individual. My emphasis is, rather, on the element of desire that moves the person from one part of the semantic/social space to the other. This desire is inner; it belongs to the inside of a person, or to the inner skin, seen here as the opposite of the outer skin. The distinction between skins is not just one between roles or categories; but also between aspects of the self, and the body is not so much a metaphor for the spirit as it is a set of metonyms for the person. And the fact that desire is at work in these metonyms is shown by the point that it is always the outer skin that is bad and also removable. The inner skin, the desire, the ideal, is good, beautiful, and young. Folktales thus evince a fantasy of desire, one that in their daily aphorisms people may wryly recognize as impossible. As the Melpa say, "We will not shed our skins," and yet, as a Melpa woman (Rumbukl, the wife of the big man Ongka) once humorously told me, "Only my skin is old; inside my *noman* is young and fresh *[kundil ninim,* applied also to cool, spring water]." Ideally, a good state of the *noman* can influence the skin and make it good, but Rumbukl's aphorism recognizes that this is, in turn, emcompassed by another condition of embodiment: mortality.

Skin, Decoration, Clothing

The outer skin of the skin changer functions in folk tales somewhat as clothing does. Earth paints applied to the skin also alter the appearance and signal, for example, festivity or mourning, along with other appropriate items of "costume." In Hagen orange, yellow, or white mud is used to mark mourning and is smeared not only on the face and body but over the hair and, in the case of men, over the beard as well. Hageners draw attention to the dry, flaky appearance and "feeling" of the skin that is produced by this means, and it is possible to compare this effect with the skin of the recently dead person, suggesting that it is an attempt to identify with the discomfort and decay of death, a practice of "death couvade" lasting for the period of the funeral. Participants are always glad to wash off the mud later, after they have made their public showing as mourners. The mud, as a "dead skin," is thus washed off, revealing the "good skin" underneath. Oil and paints applied to the skin as decoration function in the opposite way, enhancing the wearer's healthy appearance and vivacity, as do the many forms of shell decorations, marsupial furs, and bird plumes that dancers attach to their bodies, setting up numerous metonymic relations between themselves and the objects they wear. (The process of association or categorization is similar to that whereby in New Ireland the term *tak*, or "skin," refers to the surfaces of the land and of sculptured images as well as to the human body [Küchler 1992].)

Decorative costumes, from one viewpoint, are an outer manifestation of the inner state of dancers (M. Strathern 1979). They correspond both to what I have called desire and to the moral state of those who wear them. From another perspective the wearers draw to themselves the power and beauty of the items they choose to place on their skin. For the Melpa and the Wahgi peoples the conjunction of these two spheres of influence produces the overall effect of their dancing performances. A kind of dialectic is involved. Participants may spend resources on their costumes, but, if their inner state is unfavorable, even expensive items will not be beautiful. On the other hand, a good inner state should enable them to secure fine decoration. From either side of the equation we can see that the inner state is seen as the dominant factor. In practice, however, this inner state is one that is only speculatively deduced from the perceived success of the dancers. "Inner state" is actually thus in the "outer state" of the eyes of the beholders.

O'Hanlon has analyzed the process of assessment of dancers among the North Wahgi people (1989, 111 ff.). Such assessments are usually post hoc and not voiced during the actual dancing displays, since to do so would probably cause a hostile reaction. O'Hanlon points out that in the first place there must be *many* dancers; otherwise, the group as a whole will appear weak. The dancers should also be tall, straight-backed, and not too old, and their flesh should be firm and full (this is the theme of having a "big skin," indicative of the grease just below its surface, as we saw earlier for the Paiela: it is the equivalent of life force as against death). Their legs should not tremble but should tread the ground firmly, and they should display confidence. Both drumbeats and the men's singing should be resonant and full. Their headdress plumes should sway backward and forward vigorously. All of these criteria reveal that dances are festive occasions that take on the character of political displays of strength.

O'Hanlon argues that surface qualities rather than color as such are important in Wahgi assessments, although he reports an emphasis on the red/white/black triad, which is also found in Hagen and is symbolically significant (A. J. and M. Strathern 1971). Red (*bang* in Wahgi, *kund* or *kundi* in Melpa) can have both negative and positive qualities, and its connotative fan appears to be the same in both languages. We have to recognize that the same color may in different contexts carry different associations and that color is crosscut by further dimensions of aesthetic assessment. O'Hanlon finds for the Wahgi that a dominant axis has to do with appearances that are "glossy" (or "bright," as I put it for the Melpa) as against ones that are "matt" or dull, dry, and flaky (= dull) (1989, 118). The accent on glossy surfaces is consistent with the practice of rubbing fat and oil on the skin and of consuming pork fat to make the skin glow. As O'Hanlon notes, it is arguable that "in gorging themselves upon their own autogenically produced substance in front of thousands of spectators Wahgi men realize a dream of clan self-sufficiency" (120). If he is correct here, the Wahgi men enact in an external circuit of pork consumption what is elsewhere played out in the theme of an "internal grease cycle" involving the consumption of parts of human flesh. Wagner (1967) for example, has noted the importance of the consumption of pork fat among Daribi men for the re-creation of their own vital substance, equated with the sperm by which they reproduce themselves sexually. The Daribi, however, also appear to have practiced the consumption of the flesh of corpses, thus directly absorbing into themselves the substance of their relatives and recycling it through themselves. Endocannibalism of this kind may reasonably be described as contributing to an internal grease cycle (see A. J. Strathern 1982). Pigs are also widely regarded in Melanesian narratives as historical substitutes for the consumption of human flesh (see, e.g., Stürzenhofecker 1995).

While the Wahgi might thus seem to be concerned with the augmentation of substance, an aesthetics of physical strength (for males), and an emphasis on "fat" as a marker of substance and strength, O'Hanlon's analysis also shows the importance of a moral dimension that is at work. It is this dimension that brings us back again to the mindful body as opposed simply to the body of substance. Essentially, all kinds of moral transgressions may lead to a failure of a dance display. That a group is numerous or small is seen as due to its own moral actions in the past. Fighting against a "brother" group, for example, prevents men's skins and decorations from looking good. At the heart of this attitude is the deprecation of treachery. A disgruntled traitor to a group may secretly give away sorcery substance to its enemies, and these can then wreak havoc. The effects of such treachery can be reversed only if it is confessed, if the "talk is thrown into the open"

(O"Hanlon 1989, 127). Men go into a war magic house before dancing in order to make general confessions of anger they have held against their fellow dancers, and, if their decorations still appear shabby, they may be admonished to confess further ill feelings, since their hidden grudges are still preventing their bodies and adornments from looking impressive and beautiful. Nothing could show more clearly the intimate interplay between morality (mind) and successful display of the body and in this regard, again, the Melpa and Wahgi patterns are at heart identical. O'Hanlon sums up the theme aptly when he writes of the "authenticatory role" of bodily appearance (134). Equally, he remains attuned to the empirical processes in Wahgi life and history when he notes that, although in theory assessments of the body should provide "political verdicts," in practice there is always room for ambiguity and disagreement. He questions Biersack's analysis of "growing the skin" among the Paiela not in terms of its basic logic (which, as we have seen, applies also to the Wahgi) but in terms of the impression she gives that certainty of evaluation is attained. It is probably true to say that Biersack was more concerned with the code than with practice, and this possibly because the puberty rites she discusses had become a thing of the past, whereas O'Hanlon is dealing with events he directly observed and in which he participated. His observations also show that bodily movements and aspects do not always produce an overdetermined and powerful effect through their simplicity, as Connerton has argued (see chap. 2). They indeed aim at this effect, but, since interpretations vary, the aim is not invariably attained.

A striking feature of the Wahgi and Melpa materials is that the moral state of the dancers affects putatively not just their skin but also the decorations—or "clothing"—that they wear. This fact illustrates my proposition that such items are metonyms for the person, or, simply put, are parts of the person. The dancer's inner state, skin, and ornaments form a single field of force. If this is so, we should expect to find that such a basic orientation would apply also to contemporary contexts of change in which European clothing is worn. While there is a plethora of materials on the significance of "traditional" items of clothing, materials on contemporary practices and their meanings are more fragmentary.

One major influence on patterns of change has been the activity of Christian missions. From earliest colonial times these have tended to set themselves against traditional forms of dancing and decorations on grounds that these were sinful, leading to promiscuous behavior. It is interesting to note here that the "battle for the soul" was often expressed as a "battle for the body" in terms of its clothing. Moreover, missionaries were perhaps more in consonance with Melanesians than they imagined when they constructed a relationship between clothing, the person, and moral states. They attacked as "sinful" the most highly valued forms of decoration and display, on the grounds that these expressed or would lead to promiscuity and wrongdoing. If I am correct here, while their specific evaluations ran counter to the people's established values, their logical code of interpretation was sufficiently similar for the people to be impressed and to take them seriously. Indeed, this may be true of wider fronts of activity engaged in by missionaries. Believing in spirits, they relabeled them as evil and satanic rather than good and beneficent. Believing in the moral/magical significance of clothing, they urged people to take up Christian garments, which would reflect introduced values.

One drive, of course, was to cover up skin, since this was held to present the greatest dangers of sexual temptation. Another seems to have been to dress both sexes in clothing that itself was lacking in attractiveness: hence "Mother Hubbard" blouses for women and long, shapeless trousers for men. Baptismal clothing more clearly shows the same inner-outer symbolism that I have remarked on already. White is usually chosen as the color of clothing, and it stands for the washing away of sin and the new life of conversion to Christianity.

We are rather lacking in data on the overall symbolism of introduced forms of clothing in Melanesian contexts. Such clothing stands for modernity, the abandonment of the old ways, urban life, and so on. This does not necessarily imply that older meanings or codes have ceased entirely to operate. A striking example is given, in a context of ambiguity and contested meanings, by Deborah Gewertz (1984) in her account of her struggles to become accepted as a field-worker and a person among the Chambri people. Gewertz wished to have permission to enter the men's houses, which were otherwise prohibited to women. The men at first refused then relented in the face of her demands. Among themselves the people developed a hypothesis that she was "probably not a woman at all, but a strange creature who grew male genitals upon donning trousers" (618). They also thought that her husband at the time was a "feminized male," because of his secondary role in the fieldwork process. And they decided that she had bought, rather than given birth to, her only child.

At first Gewertz interpreted her classification as a kind of compliment, later considering that in fact it had made her anomalous, denying her a true or normal human social status. A necessary background to her interpretation is the Chambri view of the person, composed of affinal and agnatic relationships, and the necessity to maintain these, along with an uneasy sense of gender relations in which "women are treated as inferior by men, who nevertheless believe them to be superior" (Gewertz 1984, 626). Men do not wish to be indebted to women. At initiations, scarification and bloodletting are designed to remove the "deleterious effects" of mother's blood. Men denigrate their wives while attempting to recompense their affines for the gift of a wife. All of these points indicate that a simple relationship of equality with a woman is something that Chambri men find hard to envisage.

Gewertz does not come back to the problem of how she was defined at the end of her essay. Yet it is necessary to do so in order to explain further the logic of the "bodily" interpretation of her that the Chambri made. This interpretation testifies to the bodily definition of the person and the necessity for that definition to have a sexual component. It equally indicates the idea of the "magical power of clothing," such that it can generate a change in the person's body. Gewertz's reference to this theme seems not quite complete, however. What did the Chambri think happened when she took her trousers off? They clearly had a physical/sexual definition of the person that did not allow that a female could sit in the men's house. To let her in, they had to redefine her as temporarily male, attributing the power of making her so *to her trousers*, an obviously male piece of clothing. The trousers, I suggest, were seen as a kind of magical and removable second skin, which she put on when she wished to enter the men's house and took off when she reentered other contexts, in the same way as we have seen skin changers narrated as doing. It is this aspect of Chambri ethnotheory, then, that needs to be explored further.

If I am correct in this speculation, it gives us potential insight into the adoption of European forms of clothing generally. If we see these as having been interpreted as "extra skins," embodiments of magical force and strength that could be put on and taken off at will, it is easy, in the words of Julia Blackburn, to understand "how a conquered people often imitate the military disciplines, the style of dress, and the words of command which they have seen and heard used by white men in an attempt to adopt the power of these unfamiliar rituals (1979, 25). Accounts of first contact in the New Guinea Highlands abundantly confirm the idea that the local people saw the incomers' bodies as special loci of power and also danger to themselves. Blackburn quotes the Berndts's descriptions of events among the Kamano and their neighbors in the 1930s. When they were first shown cloth they rubbed it with magical leaves and swallowed them. "When they met men who had actually seen the strangers, they rubbed the men's eyes with these leaves and ate them. The leaves, they believed, had absorbed some of the new power" (40).

Clothing, also, was held to contain aspects of such power. European cloth was called, for example, *mukl mbal*, "the male apron from the sky," by the Hagen people, who associated the first European explorers in their area with powerful light-skinned Sky People in their own mythological traditions of remote origins. Another early term, perhaps more playful, was *kor wamb-nga kui tina*, "the white marsupial of the spirit people," a phrase stemming partly from the fact that in mythology the Sky People are the owners of marsupials in the high mountain forests. The term *kor* was prefixed to the name of objects for which a homology or analogy was found in the indigenous culture. Steel axes were called *kor rui*, "spirit axes," and the indigenous stone axes relabeled as *mbo rui*, "native axes": this reclassification amounts in itself to an indigenized colonial way of seeing the world, part of the development of a "colonized consciousness." Aspirations for both modernity and magical power can be fused together in the wishes that people clearly have to possess and wear European cloth. They sometimes describe the action of wearing such clothing as "turning into white people." This is the usage that underlay the rather cutting remark of the leader Ongka at the end of my first field trip, when I and my wife were changing our clothing before departing: "They are turning back into white people." The verb used here for "turning into," *rökli*, is the same word that is used for wearing clothes on the lower part of the body, as, for example, trousers, skirts, which also are clear marks of gender. *Rökli*, we might suggest, refers to clothing that has a close association with gender. If this is so, the Melpa case might also help to illuminate the Chambri men's assessment of Deborah Gewertz discussed earlier.

The same verb, in fact, is used as a general marker of identity change. A man who dresses as a woman is described as *wuö amb raram,* "a man who behaves like a woman / turns into a woman." A change of clan identity is expressed by the same verb, as is a change in lifestyle or self-identification in ethnic terms: *kundi raram,* "he/she behaves like / turns into a white person." More neutral in its implication is the verb *pöki,* "to cover," "to pull over the head," used to speak of clothing worn on the upper half of the body, such as blouses, shirts, pullovers, jackets. In skin change stories both verbs may be used in tandem: the person takes off / sheds the old skin and puts on / pulls on *(pöki)* the new one, thus "turning into / behaving like" someone different *(rökli).*

An implication of usage here is that one identity does not fully replace the other but, rather, conceals it. Andrew Lattas has pointed out that the "masking" of identity is often an important feature of indigenous practices and narratives and provides a vehicle for the presentation of subversive truths and alternations within narrative traditions themselves (Lattas 1992a, 12). He elaborates the overall theme of identity and change further in his detailed essay on the Kaliai of West New Britain (PNG), entitled "Skin, Personhood and Redemption: The Double Self in West New Britain Cargo Cults" (1992b, 27). His title is built at least partly as an echo of a pioneer work by Michel Panoff on the Maenge, also of West New Britain (Panoff 1968). Panoff's essay points out, with remarkable attention to nuances of meaning, that Maenge concepts of the self, including what we might translate as spirit, or shadow, are all materially based and have to do with inner and outer aspects of the body, including the skin. Lattas deploys this theme in relation to social change and the people's desires to alter their identities in answer to the imposition of colonial control. In this context skin is given maximum semiotic force. Dark skin is linked to ignorance and lack of power, white skin to knowledge, light, empowerment. Dark skin is blamed on *bikhet* (sin). As one of Lattas's informants put it: "My thought is that my skin is my *bikhet.* My *bikhet* gave me this skin, covered me up in blackness" (Lattas 1992b, 34).

The body and, more specifically, *the skin* thus codifies power and responsibility. Here taking his departure point from Read's work, Lattas notes that moral values are expressed through the body: "To not repay a debt is to have a heavy or dirty skin, whilst the moral act of repaying a debt is spoken of as cleaning one's skin" (1992b, 35). This is an idiom that finds its exact parallels in Hagen, Pangia, and other ethnographic locales as well as among the Gahuku-Gama: "To incur an

obligation to others . . . is rendered as "having a debt on one's skin'"
(Read 1955, 266). Moral similarity and difference are expressed as having the same or different skin. An individual is signified by his or her
skin, which after death will not be seen again. The Gahuku-Gama data
poignantly reinforce (as they also preceded) Lattas's argument for the
Kaliai. Taken properly, they enable us to understand the Melanesian
morality they signify as an embodied system of ideas in its own right.
Skin is "an ontology for realizing personhood" (Lattas 1992b, 35). Such
a positive perspective is quietly at variance with formulations that suggest the Gahuku-Gama (or the Kaliai or the Hageners) should be
defined in terms of a concept they allegedly lack.

Paradoxically, however, the Kaliai themselves, like many colonized peoples, appear to have come to define themselves in this way,
and in their desire to overcome this lack they adopt the strategy of
mimesis as a means of transcending alterity (on the general theme, see
Taussig 1993). As Lattas points out:

> The discovery of the magical gestures or customs which have
> given whites their material plenty is bound up with the desire to
> shed the skin and body image of the black self. . . . The black man
> here seeks to make himself into the double of the white man. He
> seeks to become white through occupying the corporeal regimes of
> the white man, that is by entering that space of movement and
> identity occupied by the white man's body. (1992b, 36).

At the same time there is a subversive element, reminiscent of the "poor
man's protest," that is implicitly present in skin changer stories that we
have examined. In one Kaliai story, taken as a basis for a movement
known as the Opu cult, the snake as a skin changer is taken as a central
figure. Followers of the cult leader Opu collected shed snakeskins,
referring to these as shirts left behind by spirits who had gone to meet-
ings in Sydney or Brisbane in Australia. Such spirits had sprung from
the menstrual blood of Opu's infertile wife as it fell to the ground, it
was declared. They had the power to turn stones in the earth into European artifacts and buildings such as planes and banks (38). Cult followers carried snakes and stated that, when God, who at first had been
with the Kaliai, ran away from them, he changed into a snake and went
to America, where he chose a marginalized, poor figure, a "rubbish

man," to embrace and empower. The rubbish man accepted the snake, and thus the snake gave Americans all their "cargo," or wealth.

In the general corpus of Kaliai folktales the classic theme of the skin changer appears in the figure of Akrit. Akrit had a black skin that was putrid and covered with sores, but underneath this he had a shining white skin, hidden from the world, a skin women were said to desire. One day he took off his outer skin to bathe, and a crab ate holes in it, enabling women later to see through the ugly outer skin and to tear it off, revealing his beautiful skin below. Akrit then married the women. The inner skin here is equivalent to the *ano*, or inside double, of the person, which, unlike the outer skin, survives death (Lattas 1992b, 47). As Panoff argued, the "inner self" here is not a metaphysical concept as such but is "more an invisible second body" (see Schieffelin 1976, for Kaluli ideas). The *ano* also travels in dreams, where it can meet the *ano* of the dead who now have access to cargo. Dreams therefore form an important part of prophetic and revelatory rhetoric.

The Kaliai example shows very clearly the semantic importance of the theme of the skin in the context of social change in these Melanesian cultural milieux. Skin is the site of felt, displayed morality and identity (see Liep 1994, 69, on baby powder in the Massim area). Skin changer stories also make it possible for an analogy between skin and clothing to be set up. Clothing therefore becomes imbued with an aura of the magical. Within this framework we can understand in a single sweep the adopting of European forms of clothing, on the one hand, and the development of cargo cult ideas based on a dichotomous representation of the inner and outer skin, on the other. Clothing can be a mark at one and the same time of modernity, and thus a break with the past, and of "magical skin," and thus continuity with the past. Yet, clothing is the outer not the inner skin. Insofar as it is seen as the new link with wealth and power, it therefore reverses the order of the indigenous theme.

Reversals and conservations of indigenous constructs regarding the body will be explored further in the next chapter, which discusses sickness and healing practices. Acceptance and rejection of introduced biomedical forms of health care have mingled in the history of colonial and postcolonial times in the Pacific generally. What I will argue is that once again it is the concept of the mindful body that has to be kept at the forefront of the analysis. As we have seen, this *is* in a very clear sense also the indigenous Melanesian model. Yet biomedicine, in its classic, unreconstructed form harking back to the Cartesian dualism that first made it possible, is based on a sharp split between the mind (soul) and the body. We might expect, therefore, that there will be a distinct possibility for misunderstanding, reinterpretation, and conflict in the process of change in medical systems in this part of the world. "Pluralism," itself a word with multiple referents, is the overall result. Nowhere do we find absolute rejection of Western medicine, yet also nowhere do we find that it absolutely replaces indigenous ideas and practices regarding sickness and health, life and death—and these ideas themselves shift subtly or markedly in a dialectic with introduced practices and promulgations as they may well have done in the precolonial past also given the multiple passages of ideas and practices between peoples (Strathern and Stürzenhofecker 1994). Although in what follows I portray the interaction between biomedical agencies and indigenous peoples as an encounter between separate unitary systems, this is by no means intended as a general model in an essentializing manner. I recognize both the existence of endogenous pluralism (such as is found, e.g., in Mexico [Finkler 1985, 1994]) and the further complications that result from the impingements of biomedicine. One of my aims, as will be clear, is to show, however, that systemic elements usually portrayed as separate may be found together within a single cultural tradition.

Chapter 5

The Threatened Body

It is evident from the previous chapter that Melanesians have clear ideas of what constitutes health and also of what makes for a good appearance, one we might gloss as "beauty." Health can be seen as the foundation of beauty, although there are additional aesthetic standards for the latter. As we have seen, aesthetic ideas often focus on the skin as a marker of the condition of the whole body: a good skin is one that shows the presence of "grease," or fat/juice, beneath it, while bad skin is dry, ashy, and associated with thinness, sickness, and the declining condition of old age. But the color of the skin (light as opposed to dark) and the shape of its features (e.g., long as opposed to short nose) may also be important. Among the Melpa light skin is definitely preferred to dark, and light-skinned women are said to be sexually more eager than others, making them desirable partners. Women with long, straight noses are considered more beautiful than those whose noses are broad, short, or squashy in appearance. Such evaluations apply especially to the head. With regard to the rest of the body, the emphasis is on general condition, implying both vigor and health, and this is encapsulated in the notion of grease. If this is plentiful, the person is healthy; if deficient, the person is sick. Specific sites of the body may be seen as imbued with power, especially hair. A striking illustration of this is found among the Mendi people, about whom Theodore Mawe (1989) reports that a man may roll a tobacco leaf "in which he mixes his pubic hair and certain bespelled leaves which he gives to the girl concerned to smoke" in order to seduce her. Similar ideas hold in Pangia, as remarked in the previous chapter.

Throughout the region ethnotheories of the body seem to conform to an idea that the body's fluids are in a variable state of plenitude or shortage. Within this framework it may be held that it is important to maximize fluids or that the balance between fluids and their conditions should be carefully conserved. In this respect we can extend the category of "humoral system," used conventionally to refer to major thought systems of the Mediterranean, Hispanic, and Asian worlds with regard to health, to the indigenous medical systems of Melanesia and the Pacific. There is, therefore, an important "naturalistic" component, in the terms of Foster and Anderson (1978, 53), within these systems, that interacts with the kinds of "personalistic" features that have more often been highlighted in ethnographies: that is, ideas of spirit attack as the causative force in illness or of sorcery and witchcraft. The connection between such personalistic attributions of cause and expressions of morality and interpersonal conflict are well-known, and their correlations with social structure have also been canvassed (see, e.g., Patterson 1974). What has not been explored thoroughly is the interaction between personalistic and naturalistic elements in medical systems. As it happens, the theme of such an interaction corresponds to the distinction between agency and substance, which I have introduced in earlier chapters. The mindful body is the site at which the interaction is played out: it is the conjoined expression of agency and substance, and its condition is the outcome of the mutual reaction of one upon the other.

The major fluids of the body, especially blood, fat (water/lymph), sexual excretions, and bone marrow (often equated with sperm), may be seen as the site of "substance," along with bones and hair. These two, however, are often closely associated with long-term capacities for growth and fertility that are linked to the spirit world. Another major component of the body is the arena of the internal organs: heart, lungs, liver, kidneys, stomach, intestines. It is with these body parts that the various emotions are often seen as being connected, although for the Melpa and perhaps others also "shame" is expressed as being "on the skin." Emotions in turn are thought to be involved in the overall state of health or sickness of the person; hence, the internal organs are generative sites at which sickness may begin or end. Life force is generally seen as diffused throughout the body and as present in any parts or substances that become detached from it, and the connection between part and whole is seen as so intimate that harm done to the part can destroy the whole—hence the overall logic of "leavings" sorcery.

At the risk of some schematization the general logic of sickness and its counteraction can be expressed in terms of the following relations: (1) the effects of substance on substance; (2) the effects of agency on substance and vice versa; (3) and the effects of agency on agency.

These relations hold for both contracting and counteracting sickness. As initial examples of these three types of relations we can instance (1) the Hua idea (chap. 4) that *nu*, or vital essence, in the person can become depleted or out of balance and that this situation is corrected by eating appropriate kinds of food (Meigs 1984); (2) the Wiru idea that the *ipono*, or spirit of a mother's brother, may enter into the body of the sister's child and eat its heart or liver *(kolorini)*, causing a wasting sickness, if adequate payments have not been made for the child's "skin" *(tingine)* to the maternal kin (A. J. Strathern 1971); and (3) the Melpa idea that spirits of the dead *(kor kui)* look into the *noman* (mind) of a person and send sickness to the person if there is *popokl* (anger) in the *noman* itself; as also the Duna ideas that female witches can carry off the *tini* (life force) of a person in their spirit net bags in order to consume the person's essence and that counteraction must take the form of recovering the *tini* and relocating it inside the patient's body.

In all of these relations agency is involved in some sense, or substance is involved in some sense, even when we are dealing in the narrower sense with substance on substance or agency on agency. Thus, food or medicine may be used to harm or cure a person: lying behind this use is the "mind" of those concerned, the sorcerer or the curer, for example, and also the patient. This is a case of substance on substance but with agency standing behind this process on either side. Or a ritual practitioner may call back the spirit of a sick person from the spirits who have abducted it or are "holding" it by the head, as in the Melpa idiom, but in order to make his words effective he may have to offer up a surrogate or substitute for the person's body in the shape of a sacrifice of meat.

These considerations will not suffice to embrace all varieties of medical processes in the ethnographic literature on Melanesia and the wider Pacific. They do, however, give us a clear line to follow in selecting aspects of these systems for scrutiny. They also enable us to see that we can associate "curing" activities with substance-on-substance relations, and into this category fall introduced practices of biomedicine; while "healing" is linked to agency-on-agency relations and closely tied also to morality, since the moral state of the person leads to vulnerability or strength in the face of the threatening agency of spirits and the state of bad feeling within the social network. Healing in this sense operates on the network as well as on the patient's body and, indeed, can only operate on the body by altering the modality of the social network. While biomedicine operates in terms of the substance-on-substance model, introduced forms of Christianity have operated on the agency-on-agency model. (For a summary of these points, see fig. 1.)

In order to counterbalance the rather abstract effect of these formulations, I will employ a number of ethnographic case studies in order to explore further the contexts and processes of sickness and its counteraction. I take first the Gimi, whose ideas of conception, spirit, and the life cycle have already been touched on in the previous chapter.

The Gimi: Physical Logic and Spirit Action

An excellent early account of Gimi medicine has been given by Leonard Glick (1963, 1967). The Gimi, who belong to the Eastern Highlands of Papua New Guinea, live in villages, to which primary allegiances are owed, with connections also to kin and affines elsewhere. Villages are—or were—political units, between which warfare could occur, and sorcery was always suspected to emanate from enemy places. Such sorcery could be either "poison sorcery," or "assault sorcery," imaged as an attack by bands of male sorcerers, after which the victim's body was left "both mutilated and poisoned" (Glick 1967, 41), an image that might have associations of rape, as its equivalent does, for example, for the Wiru people of Pangia and among the Duna (see Stürzenhofecker 1993).

A gender element is at least noted by Glick, when he writes that women could be the victims of sorcery but, according to men, could not themselves be sorcerers, since they were "for the most part believed to be too ignorant, erratic, and irresponsible to control forces as momentous as those involved in sorcery" (Glick 1967, 41). Individual sorcerers were not named; rather, sorcery was seen as a part of collective political (and gender) processes in the wider social context. The implication is also that sorcerers were supposed to kill their victims and that sorcery as such was diagnosed post hoc as a cause of death. This would be in line with the lack of stress on finding the identity of the sorcerer and approaching him to reverse his magic, although curative ritual for sorcery was performed.

In Glick's account personalistic elements predominate in the profile of the medical system. For example, demonic beings or monsters are said to strike people in lightning storms, causing convulsions and

Modalities	Substance on Substance	Agency on Substance*	Agency on Agency
Examples of Sickness Conditions	"Poison" Sorcery Pollution	Spirit Attack on Body Parts "Assault" Sorcery	Spirit Attack on Spirit
Examples of Indigenous Counteraction	Purification, Purging, Extraction (Curing)	Sacrifice, Payment, Expulsion Spirit	Sacrifice Invocation (Healing)
Examples of Introduced Counteraction	Biomedicine	Prayer, Exorcism	Prayer, Confession, Healing ritual

*Substance on agency may also occur, as in psychotropic magic, in which putatively lethal substances were introduced into the body of a victim through food or water.

Fig. 1. Modalities of sickness and its counteraction in Melanesia

death. The bones of these powerful creatures are said to be found on mountainsides and to have valuable curing powers for convulsion attacks: an example of appropriating destructive power for beneficial purposes once its agency has been transformed (from whole creature into bones). Further, a different class of beings, *nekina,* called "trolls" by Glick, can make persons peculiar (e.g., deaf, mentally ineffective, psychotic). Certain places (pools, forest areas) are also *neki,* inhabited by trolls, and should not therefore be entered. The *neki* concept is in part an explanation for mental deviance. Persons who have "deviated" from the rules by entering such forbidden places in the environment receive a stigma by themselves becoming "weird" or peculiar. The *nekina* beings obtain some leavings of the person and perform "exuvial magic" on it, causing sickness to the person or to his or her children. Finally, a third class of agents are seen as responsible for making persons seriously psychotic. These are ghosts of the recent dead (*kore*) who seek the opportunity to possess a victim and carry him or her off to the land of the dead with them.

Glick also notes, rather puzzlingly, that, while the Gimi men express fear of contamination from the "essence" *(araka)* of female menstruation and warn boys that they will become thin, ill, and pimply if they associate with menstruating women, sickness cases are not actually attributed to the agency of human females: perhaps this is simply a part of their denial of female power in this sphere, seen also in the declaration that women cannot be sorcerers. Men do, however, use *mutana*, ritual detoxifiers made of aromatic leaves, to dispel female menstrual essence (Glick 1963, 95).

Counteraction against sickness is not confined to specialists, although such specialists do exist and are known as *aona bana*, "men of power." *Aona* is "vital force" (clearly, this is *auna* in Gillison's transcription [see chap. 4]). In dreams people (only men?) contact *aona* spirits of the environment and acquire magical capacities through their link with these. In Gillison's terms such *auna* spirits are, in fact, the result of the release of male *auna* into the forest after death. Curers therefore have spirit familiars who can help them to diagnose and treat sicknesses. There is a shamanistic aspect to their actions, since in order to contact their familiars they enter trance by smoking tobacco or chewing a special bark (Glick 1967, 46).

Glick describes the treatment procedures for some serious conditions caused by demons and trolls as "homeopathic." Thus, bits (scrapings?) of demon's bones may be fed to a patient along with a meal in order to achieve a cure for convulsions, or water in which such bones have been immersed may be poured over the patient. If a person is suffering from *neki* sickness, the kinsmen take a package of food into the *neki* place where the patient had trespassed, and after it has been nibbled, putatively by the local troll and perhaps in practice by local rodents, they feed this package to the patient. Or they collect water from a *neki* pond and pour it over the patient from sacred bamboo flutes, repositories of male power. All these forms of treatment mobilize the same power to combat sickness as is thought to have caused it and represent a kind of appropriation and redirection of an agency through substance as its vehicle. The same idea is shown in general medical action among the Gimi, in which plants with curative capacities are used and also "flesh [pork], blood, fat, pigments, fumes [e.g., of tobacco] . . . may all be eaten, drunk, inhaled or rubbed onto the body in the quest for restored health" (Glick 1967, 38). The *aona bana*'s touch is also considered powerful in itself. Such a notion of power diffused in substances obviously shows that there is a substance-on-substance component in Gimi therapeutics, but the dichotomy between agency and substance collapses here when we realize that it is the theory of *aona* (*auna*) that underlies all of Gimi therapeutic practice.

This account of Gimi medicine would give the impression that there is no particular naturalistic or humoral component in Gimi thinking, since *aona/auna* turns out to be itself a "personalistic" notion. Gillison, however, both deepens the analysis of the familial context in which diagnoses of sickness are made and introduces a humoral category into the account. During his wife's pregnancy a husband must stop having intercourse with her and must also avoid *neki* places in the wild forest, where by treading on plants he could release their *auna* into "flights of revenge against his unborn child" (Gillison 1993, 224). Interference with animals in *neki* areas may cause the animals to steal a part of the intruder's *auna* and deplete what he can impart to his child (here we have the theme of limited substance, in this case spirit substance). If he later has a child and the child falls ill, the *kore* (spirit) of the animal will attack the child. Symptoms of sickness, such as clenched teeth, are used to deduce this kind of event: "when you kill a fruit bat and cook it, it clenches its teeth at you. . . . So if your child dies with its teeth clenched, . . . a bat is taking revenge" (225). The *kore* of young or stillborn children particularly congregate in *neki* areas, seen as reminiscent of the womb, and there they devour the leavings of people and are ready also to cause death to other children. A ritual expert can diagnose which such spirits are involved and obtain magically a piece of *negina* (*nekina*, in Glick's transcription), or wild substance impregnated with the *auna* of the *kore* that has been implicated. The *negina* is placed in water, which is then poured over the patient's head; "this makes him cold and ends his sickness" (227).

Although the elements of action are all here perceived as highly personalistic, reinforcing Glick's picture, we see them intersecting with humoral ideas of hot and cold conditions. *Hot* is here also implicitly equated with *anger*, the desire for revenge by *neki* creatures who attack a victim. Menstrual blood is "hot" and must be cooled by casting it into a deep hole or a river (Gillison 1993, 178). In initiations men feed boys pieces of salted pork, which they describe as feces of the sacred flutes (also seen as giant birds of paradise) and tell the initiands that if they eat their mothers' food their skin will wither, because "women's food is hot! Women have a heat that stops boys from growing, a heat that comes from having sex and menstruating and giving birth" (263). Men bleed their noses to remove hot blood like the act of menstruating (183).

Women's stomachs are also said to be hot from grief after a loved one dies; hence, they put on clay and blacken their faces, both acts that are said "to cool" their sorrow (138). They decorate, caress, and serenade the body, and in the past, would eat it, in order to spare it the humiliation of decay and to release its *auna*. Nowadays, taking the smell of the corpse onto the skin is another way of attaching the *auna* of the dead to oneself and is a task also assigned to women. All of these contexts associate women and their blood with heat and, implicitly, with sickness.

Similarly, a sorcerer is said to apply heat from a fire to a victim's leavings, causing them to rot and decompose and thus making the victim sick. Gillison suggests that ritual acts whereby leavings are inserted into containers to rot are mimetic performances representing the placement of such items inside a woman. The sorcerer himself becomes hot in the process and must remain so to ensure that his victim dies (Gillison 1993, 314). Yet he must also avoid actual women, else he would become wet and thus cold. The details here reveal the double valency of both the female realm and the category hot. The sorcerer's magical act mimics an act of intercourse and is therefore hot (i.e., destructive). Yet, if he were to have actual intercourse, he would become cold, because his own heat would be depleted, and in this case *cold* signifies "powerless." There is clearly a complex set of gendered associations at work, all of which tend to impute the quality of danger to women. Such humoral ideas as operate, therefore, are tied in closely with representations of gender, as Meigs has shown in detail for the Hua, neighbors of the Gimi (1984; see chap. 4). In addition, we see the ideological reason why women may not be sorcerers: it is hardly that they do not contain power. Rather, they contain a prototype of power (even though men further claim that women's blood is *their* transformed semen). The male sorcerer appropriates this power by mimesis. Since he takes it from women, and his power depends on this, women cannot also exercise it on their own behalf.

The Transition to Humoral Categories: "Blood" among the Gnau

Gilbert Lewis is a medical anthropologist who has produced detailed studies of the Gnau people of Sandaun (West Sepik) Province in Papua New Guinea. In one volume he explicitly discusses Gnau medicine; in the second he analyses Gnau initiation rituals. The two volumes are held together by the significance of blood (Lewis 1975, 1980). Lewis worked in Rauit village on the south side of the Torricelli mountains, which had a population of 373 persons, divided into agnatic lineages, linked by marriage alliances notionally renewed by remote cousin marriage and transacted through bridewealth payments. A man inherits and learns spells from his agnates, but he benefits from donations of blood by his mother's people; in particular, his mother's brother must "bleed himself from the penis and provide this blood both for smearing on the sister's child . . . and for adding to a food portion . . . eaten by the child" (Lewis 1975, 36). The action of bleeding can both be like a purge for the one who bleeds and a gift to the one grown, to help him or her be healthy (girls also receive the mother's brother's blood but do not know that it is mixed with the ritual meal they are given). We see here the *nurturant* quality of blood as well as the possibility that it may be in excess or be "bad" and so in need of purging; we also see the link between blood and kinship.

A child gets part of its blood from the father, so that the father's blood is gradually diminished with each child born (the same, surely, must apply to the mother?). At first childbirth a man also secretly gives some of his own blood to his wife for her to eat, hidden in red betel nut juice. Blood is therefore an important way of establishing a bond. Blood can be given away, but it is strongly tabooed to eat one's own or one's father's blood. Yet blood that is given is vital for growth. A logic of gift giving thus underlies the elementary structure of kinship (a conclusion that fits well with Lévi-Straussian theory [see Lévi-Strauss 1969]).

The Gnau are gardeners, hunters, and gatherers, in a lowland environment that exposes them to pneumonia, bronchitis, influenza, and diarrhea, and they have suffered epidemics of dysentery resulting from indirect or direct contact with the outside since before 1939. They suffer also from scabies, head lice, tinea, leprosy, yaws, malaria, filariasis, and dengue fever as well as tropical ulcers. The Gnau themselves distinguish between "conditions" that affect only a body part and "illnesses" that affect the whole person (Lewis 1975, 131). Characteristic behavior in illness so defined is withdrawal and what appears to be self-neglect, including begriming the body "with dust and ashes" (132). This form of behavior is, in fact, a strategy: the patient aims to evade the attentions of a spirit that has made or may make him or her further seriously ill. Food associated with a particular spirit, for example, is avoided (139). The patient consciously tries to appear wretched, dying in fact, so that an attacking spirit will consider its work done and will leave. It is not the aim to encourage others to neglect him; indeed, patients are bitter if kinsfolk do not tend them (134).

A living person is thought to have a shadow soul *(malauda)*, but this is separate from the spirit *(gelputi)* that they become at death. The shadow soul does wander in sickness and may have to be guided back (Lewis 1975, 157). Formerly corpses were smoked and pieces of bone collected as relics (a man scraped parts of his father's bones as "food" to strengthen him). *Gelputi* spirits are held generally to go to the sky, where also dwell *maleg*, myth spirits of origin times. Major spirits of the latter kind preside over ranges of foodstuffs (165) and may also strike people with "arrows" that produce sickness, while also presiding over healing rituals (171). In the case of one spirit, *Panu'et*, the healing image is constructed of plants, which are specified as the spirit's heart, ribs, lungs, etc. These plants are in fact collected from the garden areas of the person who is ill (172). This is a crucial piece of information. It shows that the aim of healing is to reconstitute the substance of the sick person by association with the power of the sacred landscape to which he or she is personally attached: this is a mark of the Gnau concept of the cosmos, in which the substance (or "humors") of the person is linked with the substance of the environment.

At another level what is enacted in healing rituals is the taming and eventual expulsion of the spirit from the village. If we recognize the deepest level as naturalistic, in a sense this next level (the level of syntagm as against paradigm, we might say) is personalistic. The spirit image is constructed and welcomed into the village, placed on a platform. Elaborate songs are sung in its praise for days and nights. The patient is brought briefly before the spirit effigy at set times. Then the spirit"s image is "killed," and the spirit is thereby released and ordered to depart, thus ensuring the recovery of the patient. At this level the identification of patient with spirit is disrupted by the healing drama. Meanwhile, all participants, including the patient, are strengthened by distribution of a ritual soup, and the patient is washed and discards his or her sick role. The healing is a sacred community drama based on a combination of naturalistic and personalistic logics. Such a combinative form of reasoning is seen clearly in Gnau ideas regarding food. Ingestion of food can cause harm, but this is because, as we have noted, "spirits watch over foods. Eating the food may then single out a person for their attention, especially if it is from the person's own garden"

(Lewis 1975, 307). It is this same food that is then turned into a spirit image or else is re-ingested as medicine by the sick person after it has been bespelled. Food is medicine, and medicine is food: the intentionality of spirits makes it good or bad. This image schema is exactly what we would expect to find from an underlying "mindful body" philosophy.

In terms of pathology the most clear statements made by the Gnau concern blood (Lewis 1975, 202). The blood of an old or sick person "dies"; in conditions of diffuse pain it "flows about"; blood goes to the head and causes pain; it is let out to relieve pollution; a spirit attacks a person's knee and makes the joint swell with blood; and the people are afraid of leeches because these suck their blood. Therapy often consists of rubbing the skin with nettles to make the blood move inside the skin or of cutting the skin to let blood out (143–44). Such details suggest a Gnau "ethnoscience" of the body based largely on the distribution and condition of blood, thus giving proximate causes of sickness. Spirits attack people by "drawing blood" out of them. A hunter's blood goes into his arrow and thus into the animal he kills, so that he may himself not eat his kill (blood causing exchange again). Through sorcery blood can be heated and strike the person internally (204). There is an antithesis between menstrual blood and male activities; contact with it, for example, could cause a man to fail in hunting. (Since the hunter's own blood is thought to go into his arrow, perhaps we have a theory here of antagonistic bloods, but the Gnau men actually say that the woman's blood would flow over the hunter's eyes and hide the game from him.)

Menstruating women are themselves at risk from the attentions of male spirits, who are associated with pools and sago stands (Lewis 1980, 125). While in some other cultures we will consider (e.g., the Huli) menstrual blood is considered hot, the Gnau men declare it to be cold and therefore inimical to men's "ritual heat," which they require for the successful performance of rites. Women's menstrual cold can ruin these rites, but the men's heat could also harm the women. Such an ideology obviously explains and justifies a sexual separation and a male-controlled ritual hierarchy. But it is also seen as a form of mutual protection. Thus, a man has to bleed his penis and remove heat from himself after killing someone. Only then could he resume intercourse with his wife. Gnau ideas about blood pathology (i.e., substance) are complemented by their notion of the *wuna'at*, or vital center of the person, which may be attacked by assault sorcery *(langasutap)*. The *wuna'at* was held to be in the center of the chest. Hot stones were applied to a boy by his mother's brother at this point to strengthen him. It is the center of both thought and feeling; in trance it is turned round toward the back and/or is empty.

In another idiom this same condition of the *wuna'at* is used to describe illness (Lewis 1975, 210). *Wuna'at* is not linked to spirit or soul, but it does refer to consciousness. Lewis meditates on the embodied nature of the concept when he writes, in a way reminiscent of Onians's description of the ancient Greek idea of *thūmos:* "Wuna'at names the part of the body where are localized vitality, thought, and emotion—functions which by this shared localization seem bound or intermingled in a way that our folk concept of "consciousness" supposes a quite similar complex of involved functions sited in the head or brain." Again, "emotions and states of mind are not made abstractions but identified by verbs describing characteristic gestures, or movements of the skin or *wuna'at*" (211).

While some aspects of sickness, then, are signaled by discourses regarding the *wuna'at* and spirits, the medium through which health or sickness is transmitted is blood. Menstrual blood is powerful but may make a sick person worse. Sexual intercourse itself is hot and therefore may induce sickness. A very sick man should not be touched by men who have recently had sex (Lewis 1980, 128); for a woman it does not matter. Penile bleeding is a secret men's rite, but Lewis hesitates, correctly, to equate it with symbolic menstruation. It is an aspect of male control, purification, gift giving, nurturance. For the Gnau, then, the gendered meanings of blood and its pervasive importance for health and sickness indicate that it is the "humor" of the body par excellence, whereas in some other cultures—for example, that of the Hageners—we find a dualistic system of ideas centered on the interrelations between blood and grease. We have also seen for the Gnau the association between heat and danger, which appears also among the Yupno.

The Yupno: Hot, Cold, and Cool

Humoral systems imply the desirability of a balance between elements and equate health with such a balance and therapy with reestablishing it when it has been disturbed. This systemic feature is found very clearly in the case of the Yupno, a people belonging to the Madang province of Papua New Guinea studied by Jürg Wassman, Verena

Keck, and others. The Yupno number about six thousand five hundred people, living in a range of territories varying from 700 meters to 2,200 meters in altitude. They were brought under colonial control rather late, being first visited by an Australian patrol officer in 1936. They divide themselves into fenced-in hamlets, *jalap*, occupied by family farmsteads (Keck n.d. 41) belonging to lineages or lineage sections of dispersed patrilineal clans. Bride-price is paid, and debts connected with it cause tensions between people. A son-in-law may not sit down in a house beside his wife's parents, a rule that precludes close bodily contact between them: if this rule is broken, both parties expect to suffer from an incurable attack of swollen knees, rendering them particularly immobile in the mountainous terrain.

Bride-price is paid to the clan and linked-clan relatives of the bride and is supposed to be followed later by a partial return gift. There is a stress on paying a large amount of wealth, and the whole village of the groom contributes. The wealth is also supposed to be distributed widely to the bride's kin through a set of tallies, or reckoning sticks. A kinsperson left out will be angry and is thought later to cause illness, which usually affects the child born to the married couple (Keck n.d. 54). Because the recipients themselves typically have to pay back debts in a generational cycle from each new marriage, there are often enough hard feelings and grudges, which then are seen as resulting in sickness.

These debts and bad feelings are said to settle on the skin (*ngop*) of those whom they affect. They can affect the *tevantok*, "vital energy," of people, causing them to be ill, or "hot" (Keck n.d. 66). An individual also possesses a *wopm* (image), which becomes after death a *monan* (breath, wind). In bodily terms the person may be in one of three states: hot (*tepm*), cool (*yawuro*), and cold (*mbaak*). To be cool is the ideal condition, associated with "being in the center," being in harmony with others. To be hot means to be in pain or to be angry, to be "above" others. Being cold refers to the state of people whose vital energy has been weighed down or made cold, perhaps as a protection against becoming ill or against attacks by a bush spirit known as *sindok* (71). Only the hot condition as such signifies sickness, and therefore therapy always aims at achieving a cooling effect. Yet hot can also signify secret ritual power (72), a conjunction of ideas that is found elsewhere. Sickness is the result of the exercise of power by an agent, and power is seen as hot rather than cold. In highlands societies menstrual blood may similarly be seen as hot but also dangerous, life threatening. Contrariwise, it may also be seen as creating a cold condition that is antithetical to men's ritual powers. *Cold,* in turn, may *also* have the positive connotation of fertility, reproduction (although perhaps in these instances the better translation would be *cool*). We see here a circuit of meanings with positive and negative signs added as one spins the "wheel of meaning" a little further each time.

Therapy for the Yupno depends partly on the use of substances that partake in the hot-cold dichotomy (Keck n.d. 72). Red and black earth pigments, plants, and stones representing spirits in the male cult are hot, as are sexually inactive young people. Menstrual blood for the Yupno is cold, as are thorny, dry, stinging plants, spicy foods, and creatures of the sky such as the eagle. Anger, like ritual power, is hot. It makes the *monan* rise in the body and transfer itself in an attack on others. (For the Melpa, also, anger is sometimes expressed by saying that the heart, *muntmong,* rises up and fire enters into it, while calm results from the heart sinking down again and becoming *koma* [cool], like the Yupno *yawuro* condition.)

Cooling objects include ones that are white, water, and swamp plants, also the juice of sugarcane and green leafy vegetables (spinach), which lose moisture when cooked. Persons who have frequent sexual intercourse are also cool or cold. Hot medicine is given to induce abortion (Keck n.d. 74), and labor pains are themselves said to be hot and must be alleviated by the application of water and ferns. The birthing mother's *monan* is hot and can be transmitted by touching, which may be dangerous to others; hence, she is secluded (similarly, a menstruating woman is hot and therefore dangerous, even though menstrual blood is itself cold).

Hot thus can signify anger, pain, ritual power, and sickness. In particular, the angry ghost of a person who died with a grudge over brideprice payments may become hot and thus "pathogenically active" (n.d. 79). Old people must be cared for; otherwise, they will turn into angry ghosts when they die. (Again, there is a parallel with the Melpa, among whom a mother is stereotypically expected to become angry as a ghost if she was denied consumption of pork in her old age.) It appears that only the ghosts of the relatively recent dead are active. After a while the dead soul swims down the Yupno River to the sea (and becomes cold, we may add), or nowadays in the Christian version it goes to the sky (also cold [see my earlier remark regarding the eagle]).

Sickness is tied up with the existence of *njigi,* "oppressing problems" (Keck n.d. 93). Such problems in social life have bodily results, according to the Yupno. An offended or injured person's belly becomes hot and burns, and the breath soul, or *monan*, rises up and harms the object of anger or someone in the same kinship group. The crucial basis of therapy is therefore to discover the source of an oppressing problem and to set it to rights. In the actual therapy substances may be used, but they cannot have an effect unless the underlying problem has been addressed. The Yupno medical system thus provides a perfect example of the combination of agency and substance that goes to make up the mindful body. Agency works on agency through the mediation of substance.

A system of this kind depends greatly on divination as a means of diagnosis. The humoral theory permeates this realm of action also, making an immediate connection between agency and substance. For example, if a male patient asks for water and sugarcane, this points to an affair with a woman (here seen as cold apparently, although intercourse itself is hot) and to the hot anger of the woman's husband, which now causes the sickness (Keck n.d. 94). In therapy the same logic shows. For instance, in the sickness of a child whose case history is central in Keck's account, white lime powder was at one stage applied to the child's skin and a small heap of it blown from the child's hand as a ritual expulsion of the ghost that had caused the sickness. The white, cooling lime became the vehicle by which the ghost's heat was to be removed from the child's skin (seen here as the embodiment of its moral condition in classic fashion [see chap. 4]).

Since money has come to be a part of bride-price payments, it also is morally charged. An attack by the angry *monan* of another causes the *wopm* soul of a person to leave the body, inducing sickness, and therapy may aim at inducing the *wopm* to return (another classic theme). Christian prayers, another introduced element, are combined with the drinking of consecrated water and with the suspension of a coin from the neck of patients in a syncretistic attempt to alleviate the condition (Keck n.d. 124). The coin is then used to touch all the participants in the therapy group as a sign that they are harmonious and reconciled. The skin of the participants should transfer coolness to the coin, which then can act as a source of coolness for the sick person. The choice of money as the vehicle here is not random. Wealth always has a sacred, life-giving aspect in Melanesia. Equally, disputes about wealth can lead to anger, spirit attack, sorcery, or death. Wealth is ambivalent, but when cooled by the bodies (skins) of people it can act as a healing agent, totalizing each metonym in itself.

Such a highly charged, local form of therapy cannot easily be replaced by an introduced biomedical system. The Yupno do use the introduced system but are suspicious of it, since the practitioners are non-Yupno and the hospital, as distinct from the local aid post, is rather far away. The use of biomedicines is likely to run in parallel with attempts to handle underlying perceived problems: a cure may be seen as effected by introduced medicines *and also* may be interpreted as a sign of ritual success. The Yupno have their own specialist curers of either sex, who use cooling substances as remedies (Keck n.d. 155) and are paid a fee for "soothing," or "extinguishing," the heat of conditions perceived as physical and not necessarily resulting from an oppressing problem: biomedical cures slot easily into this niche in the system (177). Keck refers to conditions of this sort as "disorders" rather than "illnesses." But biomedicine by itself is held to be incapable of removing the cause of "real illness" because of the link between illness and morality. A healthy, cool person must have balanced social relationships (197). There is a residue, *nduara* (Melpa word *nit* [a mark, depression, cut]), from every act of wrongdoing, and this may in time produce illness. If a person steals a pig and eats it, the *nduara* from the pork will make his skin loose and mark him out, also making him sick (198). In this case, then, the wrongdoer becomes sick as an automatic effect of the act, whereas in other contexts the one who is wronged projects negative emotions onto the wrongdoers or their kin and causes the sickness.

In neither case is it the wronged person who becomes sick, as happens with the Melpa, among whom anger (*popokl*) may cause a resentful person to fall ill, and therapy depends on the revelation of such anger as a prerequisite to healing. In both the Melpa and the Yupno cases, the overall precondition for healing is the restoration of social harmony. This makes sense in societies with dense, complex exchange networks centered on marriage and the life cycle and liable to produce discontent because of the intergenerational burden of debt associated with payments. In the Melpa case, however, aggrieved persons can draw attention to themselves by falling ill and revealing their anger, an action that may be seen as directly inducing exchange partners to take "pity" on them and pay them what they want. In the Yupno case the wronged person projects anger onto a suspected guilty set of people and thus forces them to pay, a strategy more coercive and less "optional" in its implications than among the Melpa. This in turn is consistent with the optionality that is built into the nexus of bride wealth and *moka* exchange partnerships in the Melpa case. Yet again, overall, Melpa and Yupno practices coincide in terms of their ready acceptance into their system of both biomedical practices (for ailments) and Christian ideas, an acceptance that is effected only by creating hybrid forms that transform both sides of the encounter. The Yupno *nduara* concept is nowadays translated as *sin*, although for the Yupno it has a specificity lacking in the usual sense of *sin* in English.

The Yupno case also shows a perfect combination of personalistic and naturalistic ideas, acting together and in symbolic concordance within one system rather than as markers of different major systems as in Foster and Anderson's usage (1978). It thus enables us to deconstruct the intent of that classification while reconstructing it within a single emic domain. Humoral ideas are also very clearly exhibited in the Yupno materials and appear to operate more systematically than among the Gimi. They constitute the arena of mediation through substance of agency-on-agency relations. They also show a strong correlation with gender categories, since there is a general equation of *male* with *hot* and *female* with *cold*. The intersection of gender with sickness can be highlighted further by looking at the case of the Huli, studied by Frankel (1986).

Huli Ideas of Blood: The Gendered Cosmos

Keck, in her Yupno study, insists on the separation of emic from etic domains of description and analysis and criticizes both Frankel (1986) and Lewis (1975) for failing consistently to maintain such a separation (Keck n.d., 13–20). At stake here is the definition of an "illness." Frankel found, using questionnaire methods, that episodes of conditions of pain, injury, or ill health mainly did not lead to explanations in moral or social terms but were simply given a naturalistic explanation; that is, they were not referred to a personalistic world of hostile agency or to moral or emotional causes (Frankel 1986, 73). In less than 2 percent of cases were more elaborate explanations offered. Keck comments that this finding may be misleading, since it is based on the superficial encounters of a questionnaire survey (and, we may add, Frankel was also known as a doctor); contradictory and various explanations tend, in fact, to be given for conditions, but the simplest answer to an out-sider might be *bamu*, "for no reason" (Melpa use this answer as a first line of defense against anthropologists, incidentally); and case histories must be followed diachronically. Most conditions may begin as ail-ments, which are reclassified as illnesses only when they become seri-ous; serious causes are then sought for them. Another point here is that the Huli have been extensively missionized and would thus be unlikely to refer to categories of explanation from their indigenous context in a casual encounter with a research worker, such as may have been the case during Frankel's survey (rather than in his more intensive partici-pant observation). Finally, the existence of aid posts and familiarity with their ways of classifying conditions could also influence Huli glosses regarding sickness conditions.

If we reformulate this debate in my terms, it is evident in any case that naturalistic explanations are likely to be *linked* with personalistic ones and that naturalistic forms of explanation may be a part of a humoral theory that is actually quite distinct from the biomedical pic-ture of the body. This latter is, in fact, the case. The movement of blood within the body is conceived of in broadly humoral terms; there is a concern with hot and cold conditions; and objects lodged within the body are thought of as moving around over long periods of time and causing sickness, which may have to be met with social payments of compensation. The Huli physical body is thus also a site of moral, social and personal value judgments, whether or not a condition is attributed to a personalistic agency as a cause.

This point can be seen most clearly in the case of two linked cul-ture-bound syndromes, *kuyanda* and *agali*. Both have to do with the dangerous or polluting aspects of female blood. Huli traditional society was marked by a rather strong version of sexual segregation, delayed entry into marriage for men, and ideas of menstrual danger. With *kuyanda* the idea is that, "if the child swallows the mother's blood [at birth], this blood is said to settle in the child's chest, and as the child grows, so the blood grows within it as an amorphous parasitic mass. This blood is the *kuyanda*" (Frankel 1986, 101). Frankel compares the *kuyanda* to a leech (109), an emblem of greed. Persons who grow up with a *kuyanda* in them become covetous of other people's food and can cause *lingi* sickness in people by looking at them and swallowing their saliva (140–42). *Kuyanda* and *lingi* thus amount to an embryonic theory of witchcraft (comparable ideas are found in Enga with *yama* [Bulmer 1965], Wiru with *pōi nokorikako* [swallow spittle], and Melpa with *orlomung peng ndui* and *kum* [A. J. Strathern 1984]). The condition can be diagnosed only by women, and, as these are mostly churchgoers, they are nowadays reluctant to do so openly. In a case history given by Frankel, one woman thought her daughter's respiratory problems were the result of *kuyanda* and that the biomedical treatment with penicillin could not remove all of the *kuyanda*, yet she herself would only pray for healing while hoping that her unbaptized husband might arrange for a ritualist to remove the *kuyanda* properly. As a child grows up with a *kuyanda*, there is a danger that this will burst and cause sickness if the child is hit. A mother deters her son from marrying a girl thought to have a *kuyanda* because when he beats her (note the expectation) and it bursts and kills her, he will have to pay a heavy compensation in pigs. Attribution of *kuyanda* thus acts as a stigma (Frankel 1986, 112). We may therefore suggest that a mother will not declare her child to suffer from *kuyanda* unless she is compelled to do so by circumstances, and most attributions of the condition are likely to be post hoc. We do not know enough about Huli women and their birthing practices, however, to be sure of this point.

Agali is an even more salient cultural category, and men are held to be vulnerable to it if they have sexual intercourse at any time other than between the eleventh and fourteenth days of a woman's menstrual cycle. Frankel gives a graphic account of Huli men's picture of the condition. It results from the communication of excessive heat by the woman's vagina. The heat "travels to the conjunction of the base of the penis and the colon," resulting in "a blackening of the intestines, and their twisting and tangling." Abdominal pain and diarrhea result. "The taint also travels up his spine [is a conduit of semen from the head], causing his neck to weaken and so his head to droop, as well as backache and headache." The symptoms can result in death (Frankel 1986, 106). Healing depends on cleansing the intestines by means of spells and brushing the body with leaves of plants known for their sturdiness and ability to regrow, followed by the drinking of bespelled water (108), doubtless seen as cool.

In general Huli men seem to classify women's sexuality as hot, with both positive and negative connotations. In mythological times women are said to have cooked food with their vaginas, prior to the time when sexual intercourse began. In the Huli bachelors' cult the founding myth declares that a woman's blood became the origin of magical plants used to make bachelors strong and beautiful. Yet birthing and menstrual blood are seen as dangerous and potentially lethal. Healing rituals are thus directed to cooling and cleansing and may include purges of blood. They reveal, therefore, a general humoral theory in which a balance of elements is important and *hot* stands for female ritual power, capable of causing fertility but also sickness. Huli concepts are thus like those of the Yupno but even more strongly marked in gender terms. There is also a gradation of ideas about female heat and sexuality, since the greatest heat is held to reside in the menstrual blood of an unmarried girl, which can "scorch" children (Frankel 1986, 109).

Heat appears also outside of gendered contexts. Heat is an attribute of *dama* spirits that can cause illness. Heat also emerges from wronged persons (compare again with the Yupno) and may strike down others with whom they come into contact (Frankel 1986, 144). The mention of heat in this context suggests an idea of subconscious power or anger and draws attention to the role of emotions in the causation of sickness.

Frankel notes (1986, 136) that "the individual experiences emotional states as a rising and falling of the *bu,* [life force or breath] within the body." Since the state of the *bu* also influences health, there is a connection between negative emotional states and sickness. Illnesses may be attributed to fright, sorrow, desire, anger, and spite. Fright leads to spirit loss, departure of the *dinini,* and rituals are performed to recover the spirit. Children are held to be particularly susceptible to spirit loss in this way. Desire can lead to illness when one person covets the food of another, causing *lingi,* meaning "give me what is there." Again, children are held to be most susceptible, suffering from pain and diarrhea when the desire of someone for their food enters with the food into their stomach. Desire or longing (sorrow) for a dead spouse may also lead to death through grief. One man described the feeling for his dead wife as "she stays in my lung" (and thus in his *bu,* or life force) (143). Anger may cause a resentful person to hire a sorcerer to kill another, but Huli anger does not work as does *popokl* in Hagen: it does not cause sickness in the one who experiences it.

Breath, Soul, and Mind: Huli and Melpa
Ethnolocations

Bu appears to be a dominant concept for the Huli. It is thought of as present in the liver and lung (*buni* and *gubalini*). The liver further stands for friendship and trust (compare Melpa *kaimb*, "sympathy," which also means "liver"). As Frankel points out, *bu* in a sense animates the whole body, but it is not the whole person. Rather, "life, consciousness, intellectual activity and moral sensibility" result from the interplay between four principles: *bu*, *mini*, *manda*, and *dinini*. These can be compared schematically with Melpa concepts (fig. 2).

Bodily organs as such are not mentioned, so that we might be tempted to argue that "mind" is seen as separate from "body." This is not so, however, for in the Huli case *bu* permeates other internal organs, while for the Melpa *noman* is seen as like an organ itself, experiencing emotions that can also be felt in organs such as the heart and liver and on the skin. Huli ideas on mind do seem to differ from the Melpa, laying stress on "knowledge" separate from other aspects. The Melpa, in fact, have a proximate equivalent in their notion of *man* (probably related to *manda*), knowledge derived from the father or mother. The Huli stress such inherited knowledge rather more than the Melpa do. For the Huli sickness also seems to be tied up with life force itself rather than with *mini*, whereas for the Melpa the *noman* is a crucial mediating site for sickness, and *muklnga* (breath) does not carry a heavy symbolic load. Frankel notes at one point that the Huli term *mini* encompasses "thoughts that are emotionally charged, the conscious expression of emotions *that are derived from the bu*" (1986, 84; emph. added). Breath, or life force (*bu*), is thus seen as the origin of emotions, in a way that *muklnga* is not seen among the Melpa.

There is clearly some perceived correlation between "breath" and "spirit" in both Huli and Melpa. Melpa, for example, may say of a person who is unconscious but still breathing that *"min petem"* (the *min* is still there). Yet in another vein they also say that in dreams (although the person still breathes) the *"min ökit porom"* (the *min* goes out) and wanders around experiencing the events and places pictured in the dream itself. *Min* may also overlap with *noman*, as in the usage *wuö min pei na petem* (a man who does not have a *min*), meaning not that he is

	Huli	**Melpa**
Breath, life force	bu	muklnga
Mind, consciousness, emotion	mini	noman
Knowledge, intellect	manda	noman
Spirit, soul (survives death)	dinini	min

Fig. 2. Vital principles among the Huli and the Melpa

dead or even asleep but, rather, that he is unreasonable, reckless, brave, without fear (sometimes imaged as experienced in the *min*), an idea that can be expressed also as *noman pei na petem* (without *noman*). It is clear that actual usage is predicated on a degree of overlap between categories, and this is true also for the Huli, but in locating the ultimate origin of emotions within the *bu*, the Huli appear to give primacy to breath as a conditioning feature of health within the person.

Soul loss is perceived in both cultures to be dangerous and synonymous with sickness or death. The action of frightening or startling a person is therefore risky. Playing tricks, physical violence, insults, or accusations may all be involved. Moral issues are therefore implicated, as is also liability to pay compensation. In the case of children their souls are thought generally to be less firmly attached to their bodies, and they are therefore at risk of being startled more than are adults. For the Huli, Frankel observes that, in four of the imputed cases of fright sickness among children, the condition followed a quarrel between the parents in which the husband struck his wife or actually set fire to her house (1986, 139). The child was startled and became sick as a result: if a child dies in this circumstance, the husband must pay compensation to the wife's people. Among Melpa the idea is applied further to the question of waking a person up from sleep. People are generally reluctant to do this, since someone woken up in this way is temporarily without the *min*. Ordinarily, waking up is a *result of* the return of the *min* to its body. The term for "to be startled" in Melpa is, in fact, the same as that for "to wake up," *rut ni,* although the first implies soul loss and the second soul return.

We can ask the question "Does every sickness imply a condition of soul loss for these people"? It is not easy to answer unequivocally yes, but at least there seems to be an underlying image schema that points in this direction. A processual approach is helpful here, as it is so often in analyzing sickness concepts. As a sickness worsens, so it is more likely to be thought of as involving soul loss. If "soul" is really "life force" in bodily terms, we can in fact say that every sickness initiates a quantum process of loss, and this corresponds to certain idiomatic usages; while in a further range of symbolizations the soul becomes hypostatized as the image of the person in a more disembodied sense, and we find rituals performed to attract the soul or spirit back into the body. For the Huli *bu* seems to signify life force, while *dinini* marks soul, meanings that are combined in the Melpa word *min*. The Huli perform a ritual known as *angawai* to attract a startled soul back into the body, involving a manipulation of the head, since the soul is thought to enter and exit by the fontanelle (Frankel 1986, 136). For the Melpa, Strauss discusses in detail the indigenous ritual *min kan kugli*, "pulling the soul by a cord," to heal a seriously ill person (1990, 129–32). A ritual expert (*mön wuö*) gives a bespelled banana to the patient and then determines by a form of divination known as *el mong poromen* which spirit of the dead (*kor kui*) has caused the sickness. The expert pushes an arrow through the bark walls of the house where the patient is lying and calls on a number of spirits until one is supposed to seize the stick from outside, agreeing that it is the one responsible. He further thrusts a club through the back wall of the house in order to see the spirits clustered out there and declares that, while playing in the form of wild pigs and cassowaries, they have detained the sick person's soul among them as a hostage. The expert asks what kind of pig is required in sacrifice as a substitute for the life force of the patient and promises a large pig as the major offering while ordering a small pig to be killed first.

Strauss continues:

> The little piglet is killed. A very long liana is cut, and the *mön wuö* gives one end to the sick man to hold firmly in his hand. The *mön wuö* himself takes the other end and goes out through the door of the hut with it and into the bushes at the back. Here he ties the liana to a little hardwood tree which is regarded as a bearer of particularly powerful life forces.

The expert makes a prayer to all the ancestor spirits and takes a piece of liver, considered rich in power (as it is elsewhere, e.g., among the Baruya and among the Duna), roasts it over the fire, and ties it to the end of the vine, where it is expected to attract by its smell the sick man's soul. He whistles (an imitation of the spirits) and brushes the vine with leaves, gently encouraging the soul by brushing movements to move along the vine. Finally, he enters the hut and encourages the sick man to take the piece of liver and swallow it, thus getting the soul back inside him. The expert whistles to the soul inside the patient, and, when it supposedly answers, he announces that the cure has been successful, because soul and body have been effectively reunited (Strauss 1990, 132).

A comparable ritual is performed to attract a wandering dead spirit into the body of someone chosen to be a medium (Strauss 1990, 132–34). Such rituals are always accompanied by sacrifices of pigs to enhance the connection between the communities of the dead and the living generally as well as that between the spirit and the body of a sick person or a dead spirit and a medium. Spirits have a tendency to wander into bush areas away from the settlements but to return and attack people from time to time. Rituals therefore have as one of their tasks to keep spirits in their place. Sickness, we might say, paraphrasing Mary Douglas, is spirit out of place. This idea is a leading motif among a people who are neighbors of the Huli, the Duna.

Sickness as Translocation among the Duna

The Duna are northern neighbors of the Huli people, and their rich array of healing practices, now almost entirely abandoned as a result of mission teaching and the introduction of biomedicine, displays a range of influences from the Huli themselves but also from populations to the south and west (Bogaia and Oksapmin). Their parish territories are less densely populated than those of the Huli, and they suffered considerable depopulation from epidemics of influenza and dysentery from the 1930s onward through the 1960s, as a result of indirect and direct contact with the Australian colonizing power. Like the Huli, they had elaborate notions regarding the dangerous—but also potentially beneficial—power of female blood and maintained strict separations between the sexes in spatial terms, partly to guard against this danger. Security is obtained by setting up boundaries and is undermined by their transgression. Not surprisingly, then, the exit of the soul from the boundary of the body and its entry into high forest areas, which are the realm of powerful spirits, but also of female witches, is a dominant way of imaging illness among the Duna. The pathway the soul follows is the same as that followed at death, but the ritual healer's magic is able to bring the soul back again, in exactly the same way as happens among the Melpa. Agency is at work in these images of the soul and its vagaries. The soul of a dead person, as of a witch, detains that of the living patient, and, if the separation lasts for too long, the patient will die. The ritual expert's task is to cajole the spirit into returning, by the same pathway that it has used in migrating to the forest.

The first step in attracting back the spirit of a sick person was to make a special sacrifice of a pig and ensure that blood from its nose would drip into a hollow space (*ita kuma saiya*). The flow of blood was thought of as a powerful attractant for any spirits, ancestral or otherwise, (*tama*), that might have been involved in causing the sickness by removing the *tini*, or life force (soul, spirit), of the sick person. As with all such attractants, an important element rested in the *smell* of the blood, as also in the aroma produced for the sacrifice by the subsequently cooked pork. (I suggest there is a link here with the rule that the blood must flow from the pig's *nose*, its own organ of smell, and, more remotely, with the Huli idea that pollution causes the nose to close, whereas through "an open nose flows influence and wealth" [Frankel 1986, 57]).

In a paradigmatic spell given by a knowledgeable leader, Pake-Kombara at Aluni, in the Duna area, in July 1991, the focus of the invocation was on a pair of female spirits belonging to the generic class of Payeme Ima, who in the past were thought of as inhabiting the high forest in Pake's parish terrain, Haiyuwi. The Payeme Ima is a transcendent spirit, or goddess, who is the patroness of both curing magic and of harmful witchcraft; she is also pictured in narratives as the receiver of dead souls, who accompany her back to the living when she visits men whom she favors. In an image found widely in Melanesia and elsewhere the land of the dead, presided over by the Payeme Ima, is pictured as lying within, beyond, or beneath a lake. Such lakes are found in mountain places, where birds call out and the wild pandanus nut tree grows. A translation of Pake's spell runs as follows:

Papumi and Lupumi, Batame and Peyame [names of the Payeme Ima] . . .
Where are you on your way to?
Blood flows from the pig's nose,

Where are you on your way to?
The Parotia birds cry out,
All the birds cry out;
The birds cry out,
The Honeyeater birds cry out.
Come down, down, down!
Sitting at the wild pandanus tree,
Put down a strong stone.
Sitting at the wild pandanus tree,
Put down a strong stone . . .
   (repeated)

Come down, down, from above, above.
The birds all cry out,
The birds all cry out,
Come down, down,
Come here, arrive,
Arrive at the homestead grove,
Arrive at the pig stalls,
Arrive at the leaves of the *kitala* fruit pandanus,
Arrive at the house grove, arrive at the eaves of the house.
Arriving, come,
Arriving, now,
I will give you something [i.e., sacrificial pork].

The spatial model involved here is that of a descent from the mountains, accompanied by the cries of birds of paradise, and re-entry into the compound, where the *tini* of the sick person can be reunited with its body. This ritual action is called *tini rawa ngereiya,* "making the soul sit down." Pake explained that the sacrifice of a pig is essential for this purpose. In an analogous ritual to recover the soul of a startled girl, they would kill the pig and pour its blood over taro tubers, making magic (*auwi*) as they did so. They sharpened a stick from the *kapono* tree and impaled a portion of taro and of pork on it and waved it over the girl. They would then bake the taro, and if while doing so they heard the *kiliapa* or *urungauwe* birds (parrakeets) calling out (signs of the girl's *tini* and also of the Payeme Ima herself) they believed that the girl's *tini* had returned. The taro was baked in ashes of a fire, and shoots of a *papaka* flower and of red pandanus fruit (also mentioned in Pake's spell) were brought. They scraped pieces of the taro onto the girl's shoulder and then offered her pork from under her left armpit (the armpit is often thought of as a place where souls can exit or enter the body). The ritual expert rubbed the flower and pandanus on his legs, making his ritual whistle. The two items were then planted, and when they grew well the sick person would be fully recovered (replanted, as it were).

Curers and witch finders of either sex in the past derived their power from the Payeme Ima, who also was thought of as the origin of witchcraft herself and the keeper of souls of the dead. She was said to possess those whom she favored and show them in dreams how to contact the dead, souls of the sick, or female witches who were eating the spirit equivalents of the internal organs of a sick person. Females possessed by her might run wild in the forest, and when they returned they would know curing spells (*aruatome*). To a significant extent, this female spirit is associated with the remote Bogaia area to the southwest of the Aluni Valley, and spells derived from her inspiration reflect place names from this area as well as a predominant association with water, the earth, and the forest pandanus nut tree. One such spell, given by the son of a Bogaia woman who had been a ritual expert in her lifetime, runs:

> Mother place, water place, Payeku,
> The Wape stream,
> The Urape stream . . .
>
> The place Urane where pigs root,
> Light shines on the ground,
> The sick will be healed.
>
> Pandanus nuts take . . .
>
> Mother place, water place, Payeku.
>
> Now the dry season must come
> And all have died.
> But these ones must live.
>
> Ura hill,
> Wape hill.

Healing power is linked to water and mountains and is thus represented as cool. For the Duna, as for the Huli, ritual power for killing others is represented as hot, and heat also produces sickness. We find therefore the same basic structure of ideas as we have seen for the Yupno and for the Melpa, since for both of these peoples anger is seen as both hot and a cause of sickness. The Huli and the Duna appear to have attached the idea of heat both to male ritual powers for killing by sorcery and to female menstrual powers, thus giving a strongly gendered inflection to different domains of ritually caused danger. Duna ideas are complex, however, since, as we have seen, one refraction of female power is depicted as cooling and healing as well as wealth-bestowing (the female spirit) whereas another is seen as hot, causing sickness, and blocking access to wealth (human menstruating females—yet the blood of an unmarried girl could also be considered a suitable sacrifice to the earth in the *kirao hatya* ritual traditions [see Stürzenhofecker 1995]).

All Duna sicknesses appear to have been implicitly linked with soul loss. In *kaliatawi* magic, for instance, male experts performed rituals either to break or to heal the bone joints of a person, using as ritual substances and implements pig's blood, sugarcane, taro, cordyline leaves, a fire-producing thong, and ashes. For the healing spell the pig's blood and the ashes were rubbed over the patient in a protective and life-restoring action, either to strengthen the soul *(tini)* or to draw it back into the patient, as in the previous example given. Substances were brought into play when "activated" by human agency or by spirit power. We see, therefore, that agency was pervasively implicated and that its effect was to mobilize life-giving and life-destroying powers, partly symbolized in terms of a hot-cold opposition. It is interesting to note that a similar cultural logic appears to have been dominant among the Iban people of northwestern Borneo and that it worked in a complex fashion linked with the "deep" and "shallow" meanings of speech acts (Barrett and Lucas 1993).

The Paradoxes and Challenges of Change

Fieldwork among the Duna gradually revealed a complex array of rituals employed in the past to cause or to cure sicknesses. Informants adamantly declared that since the arrival of the Christian missions these rituals had been largely abandoned and Western biomedicine adopted. For the anthropologist such a situation seems at first paradoxical. How can we explain it? First, we have to recall the coercive context of colonial action. Duna say that the missionaries sent the government first to pacify them and then brought the Bible themselves later. In this remark there is the idea that the ultimate purpose and power lay with the missionaries and their book of words. The Duna felt compelled to do as the government and missionaries said, and, once they had abandoned their sacred sites or smashed the stones regarded as the "houses," or "bodies," of their spirits, they also felt that they could not go back to these same spirits and ask for assistance against illness. In essence they made themselves hostages to the incomers and now are dependent on "outside power" to protect them against their own spirits, insofar as these are still held to exist. Yet we could not establish that the Christian churches were thought of as truly effective in combating illness; rather, the people seemed to have switched entirely to aid post medicine for their needs.

Evidence from elsewhere in the Highlands and in New Guinea generally shows that this circumstance is unusual. Yet the same evidence also shows that there are always problems of fit between old and new ritual systems. Frankel gives some glimpses into the contradictory concomitants of change among the Huli, for example. These contradictions arise from the fact that, while practices may alter quickly, the basic ideas about the body do not. This is in effect the same point that I have stressed in chapter 4 when discussing the overlap of ideas between skin and clothing.

The problems that arise are shown most clearly in the context of gender relations. From all that has been written, it is clear that for Huli men the idea of the danger of female blood "out of place" is pervasive and deepseated. The dangers of *kuyanda* and *agali* are therefore hardly likely to fade away simply because of church teaching or the availability of penicillin and aspirins at aid posts. As Frankel notes, Huli women "are in general committed church-goers" (1986, 111) and, since the church frowns on all traditional ideas and the rituals tied to them, they are reluctant nowadays to be the ones who will diagnose *kuyanda*—yet only they are in a position to do so, from their knowledge of the birthing process. Powerful dilemmas of choice are thus set up when parents suspect their child to have a *kuyanda* yet cannot hire a specialist to remove it. One strategy is for the husband to remain pagan and to hire a curer. In the past many of these curers were themselves females, and we may suggest that women would approach them independently of men. During Frankel's fieldwork he knew of only one such female curer who was still in business, and she refused to work with him because of his status as a biomedical doctor, fearing that he would put an end to her practice (112). Yet when the curer visited his neighborhood, one mother at once brought two of her children for treatment, showing that there was still a demand for the curer's skill.

Frankel's account here implies that no church ritual was able to take the place of this treatment. Equally, biomedical treatment cannot do so, since biomedicine lacks provision for removing "tumors" of this kind, which it cannot identify or locate (the same holds for sorcery projectiles, of course). Yet women among the Huli do apparently say that going to church can obviate the necessity to perform *hame gamu* magic to prevent children from being "scorched" by the heat of unmarried menstruating girls (Frankel 1986, 113). Frankel does not pursue this intriguing point further. For the men no such comforting notion seems to have been developed in relation to their fears of *agali.* The case histories Frankel gives show Christian (Catholic) men afraid that they had contracted *agali* yet feeling that it would be sinful to perform the ritual to expel it. One man's solution was to have Christian prayers and pigs sacrificed to God but also penicillin administered from the aid post. He felt that this double approach might make up for the lack of the indigenous ritual of purging the pollution from his stomach. Over time his condition failed to improve, so he eventually turned to the old ritual. When this also did not work, he fell back finally on another explanation, that the skin of a piece of pork he had eaten had stuck in his intestines (an explanation in line with the logic of *agali* diagnosis itself). Frankel also did not know how to diagnose the condition.

Men generally seek treatment quickly from aid posts, and, since the kaolin medicine they are given may help their stomachs, where *agali* is held to lodge, they may be satisfied on empirical grounds. If not, they move on to Christian prayers or finally traditional ritual. Frankel notes that Christian and indigenous ideas are particularly incompatible in this sphere of experience. The same is true in the realm of sorcery (Frankel 1986, 146), in attacks by *dama* spirits and the water spirit Ibatiri (160), and in cases in which the spirit of a deceased spouse is thought to attack the survivor (for which a ritual of protection was traditionally available) (164). In all of these contexts a dilemma of choice is set up if the *cause* of sickness is still held to be an indigenous spirit. God is certainly seen as a new kind of spirit and a powerful one who can both protect against sickness and cause it as a form of punishment for wrongdoing (165). But he is clearly not held to be omnipotent, nor is the range of healing practices available through the church broad enough to quiet indigenous anxieties, as I interpret the data. My basic hypothesis here is as I indicated at the outset of this discussion: ideas of the body have not changed fundamentally, and, whereas indigenous rituals always involved some direct action on the body itself (e.g., by purging or by rubbing substances on the skin), Christian ritual does not. We can see touches of incipient syncretism also, in the practice of "Christian" sacrifices of pigs and in prayers asking God to "wash" (i.e., purge) "badness" (i.e., pollution) out of a sick man (166), accompanied by the laying on of hands to the chest and stomach of the patient by a woman whose prayers were held to be effective (i.e., an equivalent of the female curer role). The strategic incorporation of Christian ideas is seen also in the sphere of morality. Anger may now be said to bring on sickness; pastors preach against anger, therefore, and urge people to obey them, on penalty of God's displeasure. Women tend to blame themselves for their "bad thoughts," while husbands similarly attribute their wives' illnesses to their disobedience (171). We see in all these examples that Christianity is not simply something imposed; rather, as far as possible it is worked into the strands of social life. Yet the problem of the definition of the body does remain.

For the Duna we might add that logically we would expect the problem of the definition of the soul, or life force (*tini*) to remain, since so much of Duna medicine for serious sickness was concerned with this. For the Aluni people, at least, we could not establish by fieldwork in 1991 that the Christian church services were used for healing purposes so much as has been seen for the Huli. Rather, everyone stressed that aid post medicine was the answer. In part this may be the result of historical factors: perhaps the Baptist missionaries who came to Aluni themselves did not stress healing prayers as such. Another factor seems to be involved, however, and that is the attitude toward biomedicine itself. This attitude represents an entwinement of pragmatism and belief in the magical power of introduced technology. Medicine *is* magic in this conceptualization. Its administration may not be accompanied by the same elaborate rituals as were used in the past, but its power (no doubt reinforced by its general success) is seen in magical terms. And, if it works, it *must* be able, by indigenous logic, to protect against spirit attacks and/or to recover the *tini* of the patients. If this interpretation is correct, we can see that pragmatism may in fact lend itself to the *conservation* of indigenous ideas at a deep level coupled with the *abandonment* of practices at a surface level: exactly the process that characterizes Duna responses to change in general. The strategy is not entirely foolproof. Significantly, the one condition that medicine does not protect against is held to be witchcraft, and anxieties about witchcraft have significantly increased over time, especially since diagnostic rituals and therapy against it have been abjured, and neither secular nor religious leaders will allow them to be reinstated. The explanation here seems to lie in the sphere of gender relations and men's anxieties regarding both female sexuality and female desires for the consumption of pork, previously appropriated in a more exclusive fashion by collectivities of men (Stürzenhofecker 1993).

The Duna case, then, indicates that a change in practices does not necessarily signify a change in basic ideas, and this may serve to modify the meaning of the term *pluralism*. Indigenous and introduced ideas may be "folded" into one another in complex ways, yet certain definitions of the person in terms of both mind (soul) and body may remain remarkably constant, showing the resilience of mindful body conceptualizations through time. When we turn back to the arena of European history and thought about the body, we will find another context for pursuing the same theme. (For an extensive further set of Melanesian cases of "change and persistence" in medical systems, see Frankel and Lewis 1988). I should stress again that my remarks here do not imply simply a "persistence of tradition," since it is well recognized in today's anthropological writings that traditions are themselves constantly reformulated (Carrier 1992). This insight, however, does not preclude the point that in certain respects there can be a powerful continuity of ideas through time, combined with an alteration in the contextual significance of such ideas, as Maurice Bloch has elegantly argued (1986).

Chapter 6

The Biomedical Body: Configurations of Science and Gender

From Melanesia we make a return to Europe. We have been looking at the effects of biomedicine on indigenous medical systems and the awkward interactions, symbioses, and contradictions set up between systems of thought and practice in the context of colonialism. The European tradition itself contains historical elements of humoral thinking that only over time were replaced by biomedical tenets that were based on the availability of the human body for direct investigation and thus led to the growth of scientific anatomy and physiology. Descartes's philosophy was pivotal in this regard, because of the radical split he made between body and soul (mind). Descartes himself seems to have been more interested in the "mind" part of this dichotomy, but medical specialists took up the "body" part, with a new freedom to look into bodily functions and to inspect cadavers now declared empty of "soul."

Along with science, however, ideology also began to develop in new directions. Thomas Laqueur has argued that there was a transition from a "one-sex" to a "two-sex" model that occurred around the latter part of the eighteenth century. By the one-sex model he refers to the idea that females were imperfect versions of males—for example, in the fact that their genitals, otherwise homologous with those of males, remained inside their bodies instead of emerging as male genitals did. Similarity and difference were encompassed by hierarchy. Male sperm was a purified essence of blood, concocted through heat and acting as the spiritual seed or source of life. In the Greek Hippocratic picture sperm, arising like froth from blood, passed to the brain and thence back through the spinal cord and the kidneys into the testicles (Laqueur 1990, 35), while breast milk was seen as womb blood that flowed back into the breasts and became whitened (36). The fundamental character of blood is here exemplified, and we can suggest that the one sex theory also entailed a "one-blood" theory as a part of its own basis.

"By around 1800," Laqueur writes, "writers of all sorts were determined to base what they insisted were fundamental differences between the male and female sexes, and thus between man and woman, on discoverable biological distinctions, and to express these in a radically different rhetoric" (1990, 5), which was founded on a notion of "radical dimorphism." The old idea was that males possessed more heat than females: this was now stressed in the idea that men had catabolic cells, which spent energy, while females had anabolic ones, which conserved it. Men were therefore passionate and quick, while women were passive and slow (6). Such "gender" differences were therefore now held to depend on "biology," so that biology in turn became the justification for gender roles themselves. Sex itself became more fixed, and the kinds of androgynous images of Christ remarked on by Caroline Walker Bynum (see chap. 3) could no longer be upheld. In accordance with the new idea of women's "sluggishness" the old view that conception required mutual orgasm was repudiated. It is obvious that "radical dimorphism" in this sense was simply a way of newly recreating a hierarchy and this time one purportedly based on fixed rather than fungible biological differences. Culture was now "derived" from the body rather than being consciously "read into it." As Laqueur puts it, "two sexes . . . were invented as a new foundation for gender" (1990, 150). One concomitant was that the divide between "biological sex and theatrical gender was greatly sharpened," in the name of skepticism. Such an "empirical" viewpoint was a part of a much larger change: the collapse of the hierarchical cosmos of correspondences between the body, society, and the deity, and their substitution by the idea of a universal, undifferentiated "nature" (151), of which "sex" was now a part.

Laqueur argues that the context for these changed ideas was not simply scientific knowledge but, rather, politics, and gender politics at that. Arguments about the sexes also reflected arguments about their sexual powers and were rhetorical ways of defining, controlling, or constraining power. Laqueur's argument is not that a monolithic view of sexual and thus social difference came to prevail but, rather, that the terms of the argument were secularized and physicalized. The body was not based on hierarchy but hierarchy on the body. He insists that scientific discoveries accompanied the new interest in the body but did not in and of themselves create it. And he recognizes that two-sex thinking did not entirely displace the "one-sex" model, just as humoral thinking in medicine has persisted into the biomedical era. Nevertheless, there was a change in the form of ideology, and the same rhetoric was involved in arguments regarding race as was implicated in those regarding sex—for example, that "the uterus naturally disposes women towards domesticity" (Laqueur 1990, 155) or that, as John Locke asserted, men dominate women simply because they are abler and stronger (156). Penis and vagina similarly became opposites, not inverse mirror images of each other—again, not simply because of a change in knowledge but because of a shift of emphasis.

Laqueur points out in fact that the two-sex model was created not through but in spite of new scientific discoveries, since these pointed to fetal androgyny and parallelism between the penis and the clitoris (Laqueur 1990, 169), potentially resonating with the old homologies of Galenic medicine. Yet other findings, such as that of the different but complementary constitutions of the egg and the sperm, dating from the mid-1650s onward, gave credence to the two-sex model: "sperm and egg could now stand for man and woman" (171). Conception became like penetration, in a new synecdochic view of natural correspondences, and plants themselves were also "ennobled" through granting sexual terms to their reproductive parts (172).

Arguments about women's bodies and their dispositions were used both to challenge and to reaffirm patriarchy (Laqueur 1990, 195), especially after the French Revolution, which created a new problematic for the constitution of civil society, including the place within it of the sexes. In one argument women were implicitly excluded as subjects altogether from society, since they were located entirely in "nature." In Rousseau's scheme sexual difference even became the reason why women should not receive the same education as men (200). Others argued, again putatively on the basis of biological characteristics, that women as the gentler sex had a greater moral aptitude than men and were therefore better, not worse, fitted for leadership. In a bourgeoisification of women they were also declared passionless and therefore less likely to be subject to the sway of sexual desires than men (and less in need of so-called natural outlets, accordingly). In another version of this theme women were granted sexual desire but of a higher kind than that of men. All these different versions, as Laqueur notes, pointed to women's "bodies endlessly open to the interpretive demands of culture" (217). One set of such demands was heavily influenced by capitalism. Prostitution was seen as destroying the natural functions of women and a cause of sickness and infertility, an intrusion of commodity exchange into the world of nature and of married love. Thus, "a deep cultural unease about money . . . is couched in the metaphors of reproductive biology" (232). All in all, the European data support strongly Mary Douglas's proposition that it is social perception that constrains the image of the natural body (see chap. 1).

"Anatomy is destiny," in Freud's term, was the proposition logically entailed by the two-sex model, yet for Freud the libido was shared by either sex. He noted that the clitoris was a seat of sexual pleasure but went on to argue that it should be replaced in mature women by the vagina. Vaginal orgasm was the ideal, because it was more "female," less "male like." This was a piece of pure gender symbolism imposed on physiology, since there is no real evidence for vaginal orgasm, and thus "Freud's answer . . . must be regarded as a narrative of culture in anatomical disguise" (Laqueur 1990, 236). Freud allowed libido to women but imaged it as appropriate to the organ that was the receptacle of the male organ and its opposite as passively receiving penetration. "Cultural myth is told in the language of science" (243).

Laqueur himself takes the opportunity to reverse Freud's dictum, suggesting that the truer version of it is that "destiny is anatomy," i.e., that anatomy was made into the ideological basis for destiny. The implication here is that the collapse of the encompassing hierarchical "one-sex" model of the cosmos did not really signal the ending of cosmological thought. Rather, a new cosmos was constructed not out of "divine" but out of "natural" law, and in fact hierarchical relations between the sexes were reconstructed out of complementary difference. From a feminist viewpoint one could argue that the epistemological rupture did not indicate a break with patriarchy but only a shift in its basis, and that the kinds of projections that occurred in scientific language were just as strongly gendered as those that marked theological language previously. Laqueur's own deft distinctions between *sex* and *gender* convey the point very well: gendered distinctions were now simply constructed out of different frameworks and different pieces of evidence from those previously used. He is also attentive to the fact that both the "one-sex" and the two-sex models in some sense continued to coexist, and elements of them tended to reemerge in arguments over time.

The attribution of different structures of emotionality to men and women fed into ideological practice in a large number of ways. It was used to justify male domination, since males were said to have stronger wills; to discourage men from attending salons run by women, since to do so would make them effeminate and soft; to extol the virtues of a domestic role for women, seen as the nurturers and comforters of their children and husbands; and to associate women generally more with feeling/emotion than with thought/reason. Women's bodies also became symbols of nature as "reproduction" and in this guise were suitable objects both for male sexual desire and for the gaze of medical scientists (Jordanova 1980, 54). As Jordanova notes, medical dissection was characterized in paintings by an image of "the utter passivity [female] of the living material used and the active intrusion [male] and manipulation of the experimenters" (58). Women were not only portrayed as passive but also as "frivolous and emotional," while men represented themselves as "serious and thoughtful" (63). In the late nineteenth century we find Durkheim arguing that women are altogether less "mental" than men with regard to their sexual needs and that a woman "has only to follow her instincts to find calmness and peace" (64).

Women were thus increasingly constructed as less "cultural" than men, as less mental and more natural, meaning more "bodily." Jordanova rightly points out that much of what was written on the topic of gender was produced programmatically by a small male elite intent on laying the foundations of middle-class life, and it often bore little resemblance to actual patterns of social relations. Yet the terms of the discourse became deeply interwoven in public debate, and women's lack of civil rights was sufficient to spark feminist protest movements culminating in political changes in the twentieth century. Further, the ideas involved are still to be found in popular contemporary attitudes in both Europe and America. Jordanova herself notes that in the broadest terms gender-based arguments in medical science gave birth to "a biologism which it is the responsibility of the social sciences, including history and anthropology, to combat" (1980, 67). It is important also to note that "science" did not lead to an abolition of gender hierarchy but to a reinvention of it, hence to ideological continuity in spite of massive change in practices (see the end of chap. 5).

While women's bodies were regarded as the prime locus of nature and reproduction, it is evident that the human body in general became more and more an object of investigation in biomedical terms and, although this was driven by the demands of empirical science, it also led to a growing split between medical practice and matters to do with mind. Women were granted an "emotional body," as it were, but as emotion was separated more from reason and the *object* of contemplation by reason came to be the body itself, separate from the mind, so the idea of the "mindful body" as relevant to medical investigation was excluded from purview. It was only with the work of Freud that the connection between emotion and illness was brought back into focus, and Freud's science was also one that was heavily inflected along gender lines, as I have noted earlier. The split between body and mind, canonized by Descartes, resulted eventually in a split between "psychiatry" and "biomedicine" or between mental and physical illness. It also resulted in competing claims to the category of "science" itself.

Deborah Gordon has outlined part of the terms of this ongoing debate in her chapter on "tenacious assumptions in Western medicine" in the volume "Biomedicine Examined" (Lock and Gordon 1988). Gordon broadens the issue from the outset of her chapter by pointing out that biomedicine's practice is not the same as its theory and that it is linked to Western cosmology, ontology, and epistemology, while its own theory may claim neutrality and universality (1988, 19). Here she reiterates Foster and Anderson's time-honored observation that medical systems are always parts of wider cultural systems; they are "embedded," just as economic and political systems are (Foster and Anderson 1978, 39). Because these systems are institutionally differentiated in Western societies, there develops an ideology that they are independent of one another or that one can analyze economic or political behavior in its own terms. This is, of course, misleading, but we have to see such claims as a part of the strategies for power used by their proponents. Invocation of science is an important part of such strategies and one that has been eminently successful in helping to legitimize and expand biomedicine within the wider cultural system.

Gordon's starting point for her exposition, as was mine in this book, is Cartesian mind-body dualism, seeing this as a world view that is rather resistant to change. She also cites the puzzlement of the philosopher Charles Taylor over the dominance of naturalism, the view that we are a part of nature, even though the particular view of nature involved is one that has existed only since the time of the Enlightenment (Gordon 1988, 21). Nature in this view is seen as passive, neutral, open to the will and power of the human self to control and direct it. It is a view that permeates attitudes and permits other viewpoints to appear obvious, a kind of foreknowledge, in Heidegger's sense of the term (23). While recognizing that there is a danger of oversimplification and that the assumptions involved are now being extensively challenged, Gordon sets out the basic components of naturalism as follows:

1. "Nature is distinct from the "Supernatural": Matter as opposed to Spirit" (24).

Through this proposition illness is severed from morality and religion, as also from the theodicy of misfortune in general. Reality is defined as material and separate from spirit (i.e., mind). The mindful body can therefore no longer be the focus of medical practice, since mind (spirit) is separated from body (material).

2. "Nature is autonomous from human consciousness" (25).

By this proposition "reality out there" is separated from perceptions of it. It can be the object of study by a subject. It can be separated from the perceiving subject. In this way phenomenology is ruled out. Medicine comes to distinguish between "real signs" (e.g., which a machine may record) and "symptoms" (i.e., the patient's subjective complaints). Hence the distinction between disease (objective) and illness (subjective). Doctors are concerned with the former. Emotions can cause illness, but only the category that is "psychosomatic," seen as anomalous.

3. "The part is independent of and primordial to the whole" (26).

This is a basic premise of atomism as against holism. "Mind," which gives a holistic meaning to "body," is thus again ruled out.

4. "Nature is separate from culture" (27).

Biological universalism is given a priori status. Culture is secondary, not constitutive. Culture limits individuals, who are seen also as prior to it. Culture in medicine has to do with the patients and their (inadequate) understandings, not with medicine and doctors as such.

5. "Nature is separate from morality" (28). See 1.

6. "Nature is autonomous from society" (28). See 4.

7. "Nature/Truth is universal, autonomous from time and space" (29).

Medicine is thus conceptualized as a single pathway of progress toward (biomedical) truth. Reason is also seen as democ-

ratic, "since it is open to all." And "precision, clarity, and num-
bers" are the best tools to get at "reality" (31).

In the second part of her argument Gordon elaborates her view that
biomedicine is in fact based on a particular cultural view of the individual as an autonomous, given, sovereign entity, an embodiment of
freedom, a distinct unit, prior to society and culture. This entity as transcendent subject is seen as being able also to objectify itself and its values and thus to stand separately from them. Society is also seen as
derivative from the actions of individuals and a potential enemy to
their freedom. As Gordon points out, all of these propositions are moral
propositions. Insofar as biomedicine chimes in with them, it *is* in fact
still embedded in a form of morality but a very different one from those
expressed in other medical systems. And *nature* and *rationality* together
form the basis of a powerful rhetoric of evaluation of action. The
emphasis on autonomy goes along, in North American biomedicine at
least, with a rhetoric of rights: the rights of fetuses and people in comas
are maintained and asserted. Gordon ends her discussion with an interesting challenge: "When calling it [biomedicine] 'dehumanizing' we do
well to consider what it means in western society to be 'human' " (Gordon 1988, 42).

Throughout her discussion Gordon also notes that there are coun-
tertrends within and outside biomedicine that negate the assumptions
she enumerates. A part of her own critical purpose is to negate biomedicine's assumptions by showing that it is itself, in fact, a part of the
wider culture to which it belongs, although not in a simple hierarchical
fashion: rather, there is a dialectic of mutual construction at work. It is
important also to realize that biomedicine did not spring into being
suddenly with all its assumptions fully formed. The assumptions, for
one thing, are shared by the other sciences, and biomedicine has seen
itself in particular as one of the natural, not the social, "sciences."
(Indeed, the idea of a "social science" is one that is intrinsically contested and contestable, given the assumptions of science in general, a
point that has been made clear in all postmodernist discussions in
anthropology [see Rosenau 1994].) Particular scientific traditions and
findings themselves grew up during the eighteenth and nineteenth
centuries, and it is clear from historical accounts that the "assumptions" Gordon lists were facilitated over time by particular findings
and technological inventions. I want to suggest that the treatment of the

body as an object was driven in particular by anatomy, by the invention of anesthesia, and by the manipulative practice derived from anatomy and anesthesia, surgery.

Some clues to the situation can be found in Catherine Gallagher and Thomas Laqueur's edited volume *The Making of the Modern Body* (1987). Contributors to this volume are largely concerned with the body as the site of discourses regarding reproduction, sexuality, and gender differences. Londa Schiebinger shows, for example, that anatomical representations of the female human body gained prominence in the nineteenth century as a part of a developing discourse about natural differences, which were since the Enlightenment considered to be the basis of social differences. Schiebinger points out also that the scientists who, with putatively impartial gaze, turned their attention to the female anatomy were almost always male (Schiebinger 1987, 43). The eighteenth and nineteenth-century drive to explore anatomical difference seems to have been different from the ethos that held in the sixteenth and seventeenth centuries; Schiebinger cites here the work of the French scientist Poullain de la Barre. Andreas Vesalius, "widely recognized as the founder of modern anatomy" (48), considered sex differences to be no more than skin-deep and denied that they were derived from the humors of the body. His generic "human skeleton," derived from the male, was not given an explicit sex. Two centuries later, however, scientists began to probe the human body for a wider range of sex differences that might be seen as penetrating "every muscle, vein and organ attached to and molded by the skeleton" (53). Alexander Monro in 1726 laid down three causes that explained the special characteristics of female bones: weak constitution, sedentary life style, and procreative function. In 1796 the German anatomist Thomas van Soemmering produced a "perfected" portrayal of the female skeleton, checking his representation "against the classical statues of the Venus di Medici and Venus of Dresden" (58). Others, however, criticized him for making the woman's rib cage too large and the pelvis too small—not "female" enough! In 1829 John Barclay of Edinburgh compared the male skeleton to that of the (noble) horse and the female to that of the (large-pelvised) ostrich. Finally, in the course of the nineteenth century women's skeletons were compared to those of "children" and "primitive races," facilitating a debate on the relationship between skull size and intelligence. Some argued that women's heads were larger in proportion to their bodies than those of men; hence, they must be more adept intellectually. But over time the equation between women and children came to predominate. Schiebinger shows that the drive to find sexual difference in anatomy contributed to the development of anatomy itself and to its translation into health manuals that progressively differentiated regimens of health care for the sexes.

The history of anesthesia is also bound up with gender perceptions. Mary Poovey writes in the same volume as Schiebinger on the discovery of the properties of chloroform by James Young Simpson, professor of midwifery at Edinburgh University (Poovey 1987, 137 ff.). Having tested the chloroform on himself and his friends, Simpson began to use it in obstetrics. Although the use of this anodyne was at first contested and led to a number of deaths, it was one further step in a male takeover from female experts in birthing that began with the invention of the Chamberlen's forceps. Chloroform was also more powerful than ether, giving the doctor more control over the birthing mother's body and raising awkward issues of propriety. It also, as Poovey notes, "helped transform surgery from a craft requiring speed and brute strength to a conservative practice in which careful dissection could preserve tissue that would otherwise be destroyed" (139).

The issue over chloroform is interesting in its own right, since, in the debates over its application to women in childbirth, arguments regarding nature and culture were advanced that reveal that nature was considered to be under the control of God (as culture was under the control of man). Since childbirth and women were seen as natural, it was questioned by some clergymen whether it could appropriately be brought into "culture" through technology and whether the woman's own natural experience could be overridden by the doctor's expertise. In his response to these criticisms Simpson argued that God was now empowering men to relieve women's pain and that God first used anesthesia when he put Adam to sleep in order to extract a rib from him and produce Eve.

Continuing in more medical terms, Simpson argued that, even without the benefit of the woman's own words, "a doctor could read his patient's silenced body" (Poovey 1987, 140) and an anesthetized patient would not resist the insertion of the doctor's instruments into her "maternal passages" (141), thus making the mother more passive but the birth itself more safe. Ambiguity nevertheless continued to surround the debate and the effects of anesthesia, since chloroform was held also to incite the sexual passion of those who took it. Simpson himself professed skepticism on this point but urged that, to preclude such

excitation from occurring, a heavy dose of chloroform should be pre-
scribed (144). The patient would thus be made even more passive.

In addition to the argument about anesthesia there was also discussion about the significance of the uterus in general for "defining
woman." Male specialists wrote in terms that suggested that "woman's
reproductive function defines her character, position, and value, that
this function is only one sign of an innate periodicity, and that this biological periodicity influences and is influenced by an array of nervous
disorders" (Poovey 1987, 146). At this time the concept of female hysteria accordingly came into vogue, and Poovey comments: "Representing woman as an inherently unstable female body authorizes ceaseless
medical monitoring and control" (147): a medicalization of women as
such via their reproductive functions.

Poovey's theme is one that is taken up and put to powerful use by
Emily Martin in her well-known work *The Woman in the Body* (1992).
Martin argues that a dominant picture of the body as a machine,
shaped in the machine age of industrialism, underlay medical practice
from the nineteenth century onward. In the context of reproduction the
uterus is the primary machine, and the doctor with his forceps is a
mechanic who fixes it (Martin 1992, 54). Martin goes further and suggests that by this metaphor reproduction is treated as a form of (fac-
tory) production—thus menstruation may be seen as failed production and the "efficiency" of giving birth is measured in time and
motion terms (59), while the uterus itself is seen as a machine that produces babies by work (the application of force against resistance). Uter-
ine contractions in the first stages of labor are seen as involuntary, separate from the woman's own will, and yet the woman may be urged
herself to "push." The doctor manages the whole process by seeing that
it occurs within a certain time period, namely, twelve hours. There is
almost a valuation of caesarean versus vaginal delivery, which emphasizes the controlling, and not just the managing, role of the doctor, in
fact (64), with the result that the caesarean baby, more a "product" of
the doctor than of the mother in a sense, is seen as "more perfect" than
a child produced through the vagina: a triumph of male culture over
female nature.

Schiebinger (1989, 104–12) has traced the decline of the midwife in
Europe since the seventeenth century. Midwives were semiliterate
senior women, paid a small fee for their services, whose craft came
under pressure of criticism with the professionalization of activities by
male medical specialists. Barber-surgeons, for example, formed them-

selves into guilds already by the sixteenth century in England, and in 1745 surgeons separated themselves from barbers, raising their own status. In 1616 the Huguenot Peter Chamberlen petitioned the king to allow the midwives of London to form a guild, but the attempt was rejected by the Royal College of Physicians. By 1642 the regulation of midwives passed into the hands of surgeons, and there was also increasing competition from men as birth attendants. Men invented new tools for birthing and refused to share these with the midwives. Midwives replied by arguing that the role belonged to them according to the "natural order of things" (109), but, increasingly, male obstetricians were hired by those who could afford them, while midwives were left to deal with the poor. Along with their decline there seems to have been also a decline in knowledge of fertility control on the part of women in general. Women thus "lost control over their own bodies" (112), while the specter of possible male sexual impropriety was also raised.

Loss of control over the body goes along with the suppression of meaning in illness and the development of scientific biomedicine, in which the body becomes more and more a passive object. Connected with this process is the increasing separation of "medicine" from "food," so characteristically associated together in humoral systems that enjoin a balance of elements, to be controlled at least partly by the patient or sick person himself; and the increasing professionalization of medicine itself, resulting in an enlarged gap in knowledge between the ordinary person and the specialist doctor. There is clearly, as Foucault, pointed out, at least a homology between state control in general and hierarchical control in the management of illness, especially mental illness, through which the two parallel institutions of the prison and the asylum developed. As Kirmayer, quoting Sullivan, has noted, "the real dualism in modern medicine is . . . between the physician as active knower and the patient as passive known" (1988, 60). As a corollary, "disease" (i.e., what is wrong with the biological machine), comes to take precedence over "illness" (i.e., the patient's phenomenologically felt reality), and the category "psychosomatic" comes to acquire a derogatory sense. Emotional concomitants of illness are also treated as intrusive and irrational, leading to patients' "noncompliance" with treatment. In contrast, the newer biopsychosocial approach within biomedicine attempts to reunite considerations of mind and body in relation to sickness and to acknowledge what Kirmayer has called "the body's insistence on meaning." Concomitantly, there is a shift from a focus solely on "curing" to one that also expresses "caring." Kirmayer also notes that psychosomatic medicine may perhaps fall into the danger of the Cartesian split, and he argues, from a radical and critical standpoint within medical anthropology, that in order to escape from the epistemological impasse "the exploration of alternate epistemologies and conceptions of the person is a pressing concern" (83). He echoes, incidentally, the gender bias of European culture by linking knowledge, or reason, to the male sphere and contrasting it with "women's attention to the bodily-felt significance of relationships and events" (86). Yet in other cultures this kind of hierarchical ranking of knowledge versus emotion does not exist. This gender bias can be most successfully circumvented, then, if we turn once more away from the European biomedical tradition and to the cross-cultural record of healing systems in which gender issues either do not appear or do not appear in the same way as in the European traditions and contexts (see also Helman 1988).

I move next, therefore, to a consideration of healing systems that depend on the role of trancing and/or spirit possession in the therapeutic process. Such systems bring emotion (or psyche) back to the center of the stage, but they also depend on certain conceptions of the body and the seat of life within it, which must be examined in their specificities for us to understand them. I will consider such conceptions also from the perspective of the study of consciousness and its sociogenic and psychogenic aspects in general. My focus will not be on gender but on mechanisms and processes of healing applied to both sexes. This does not mean, of course, that sex and gender are irrelevant. It simply means a shift in focus from the present chapter to the next. (For a powerful treatment of issues to do with the body and "sex" in the European and other traditions, see Butler 1993. Butler, following Foucault and Lacan, takes up an approach to the materiality of the body via the discursive limits of sex. Both Janice Boddy [1989] and Carole Delaney [1987], among many others, have pointed out that bodily symbolism may differ greatly for the sexes. Delaney, e.g., remarks that "the female body in Turkish perception is one that is relatively unbounded" and so would not fit with Mary Douglas's proposition that the body is a model for any bounded system. She notes too that in both American and Turkish culture the female body [in a sense, we might add] "is more associated with and represents corporeality more than the male" [1987, 47]. Such an argument, in turn, must depend on the meanings we give to the term *corporeality* and the level of meaning we choose to focus on.)

Chapter 7

Trance and Healing

Trance and spirit possession are known to be associated frequently with therapeutic rituals in which healing is sought for conditions of illness. The character of such healing and its precise link with trance or possession have been difficult to establish in cross-cultural terms. We are faced here with an old and familiar problem: how to move from specific ethnographic accounts to generalizations about such accounts—or, indeed, whether to attempt such a move at all. My focus in this debate will be on matters to do with consciousness and the embodiment of knowledge, which I see as corresponding to ideas of psychogenic and sociogenic contexts. I choose a set of ethnographies to discuss not in order to prove any propositions but, rather, to suggest patterns and explanations for patterns that may find resonance with other cases also. In a psychogenic vein I use concepts of mind-body healing developed by Ernest Rossi out of the thinking and practice of Milton Erickson. In a sociogenic vein, following suggestions by Paul Stoller, Bruce Kapferer, Jane Monnig Atkinson, Carol Laderman, and Janice Boddy, among others, I argue that where trance with possession is found much of the therapeutic performance consists of the presentation of a historical consciousness on the part of those possessed. As always, the term *consciousness* is problematic here. I mean by it in the first instance the communication to others of identity and intention on the part of an actor: it is the communicative context that I am most concerned to understand (for a much broader and comprehensive treatment, see Cohen 1994).

Bourguignon (1973) has pointed to differences in the incidence of trance with and without possession, linking the former to more hierarchical social contexts. While her distinctions, and refinements of those distinctions (see, e.g., Shaara and Strathern 1992), are important in general, I shall assume here that possession is based on trancing as its underlying condition and that the ability to experience trance is widely shared around the world (Winkelman 1990). Trance is therefore the basic phenomenon in psychogenic terms, and it should be possible to suggest features of it relevant to healing that can operate cross-culturally. Spirit possession, by contrast, is the locus of historical specificity.

The fundamental feature of trance is that it is a practice in which altered states of consciousness, experienced often in a layered fashion, are communicated to others. In one theory of the mind *altered* here means expanded, in the sense that what is otherwise unconscious is brought into consciousness. In another representation *altered* may refer to the adoption of a different identity: this latter formulation feeds easily into a theory of possession. In either case one problem lies in grasping the mechanisms by which alteration occurs (hence, e.g., theories of sonic or photic driving, musical rhythms, the ingestion of hallucinogenic drugs, use of tobacco). Just as interesting, however, is the problem of the coexistence of two forms of consciousness and their interplay. The latter problem is highly significant for the question of healing. Theorists usually make further ad hoc distinctions between light, medium, and deep trance. In the first of these the subject is clearly aware of more than one context of consciousness, but this awareness declines as trance deepens. Ethnographically, then, we might wish to know how to assess the trance experiences of healers or patients in terms of this light-deep contrast, but this is not easy. We may have to be content with the stated aims of the actors. In any case it is important to examine whether both therapist and patient are held to be in trance or only one of them and why.

One further problem in relating psychogenic to sociogenic contexts has to do with hypnotism. Rossi and Erickson (Erickson 1980) imply that to hypnotize a patient is to put the patient in trance and that such trance is the same as the trance experienced in systems cross-culturally. But at the least here we need to recognize differences also. Most particularly, hypnotism emphasizes the controlling power of the therapist whereas in many trance situations the alteration of consciousness is creatively entered into by the experiencing subject. That creative "entering into" may also involve the representation of the spirit world, as in possession.

I turn now to ethnographic cases.

The Temiar: Blowing Kahyek

Marina Roseman (1991) has stressed the healing qualities of sound for the Temiar, who live in the rain forests of Malaysia. For the Temiar, as for many other peoples, such healing is also bound up with their theory of "souls" in an animistic universe, or cosmos, in which the souls of people interact, blend, and differentiate themselves from those of animals, plants, and the landscape. A pervasive distinction is made between upper and lower or outer and inner souls; in humans the distinction is between head and heart souls, and the head soul, in particular, becomes unbound from the body during dreams, in trance, and in illness. It may encounter the soul of another entity, which then gives it a song and offers itself as the person's spirit guide, showing pathways for healing. A healing specialist, or medium, is one who has garnered healing songs in this way and can use them to heal others. The songs express an ability to move the heart and also the spirits. Roseman calls them "sonic icons of the heartbeat" (15), which also "set the cosmos in motion and effect the transformation of Temiar trance" (16). Fundamental to all this is the Temiar ethnotheory of "being," resting on the notion of multiple souls. The head soul is the "vital, animating principle" (25) and is a focal point of illness and of healing. It can be referred to as a "plant shoot." In trance it is said to be broken off like a snapped twig, as also when a person is startled. Temiar take great care not to startle others, yet illness may be traced to mild startling or angry words, even if spoken indirectly, the more so if accompanied by pronouncing the autonym of the person at whom the words are directed. The head soul also goes out in the voice, especially in singing (29). The head souls of spirit guides show themselves as *kahyek,* "a cool, spiritual liquid likened to the colorless sap of plants, the clear waters of mountain streams, and morning dew" (30). Mediums blow *kahyek* into patients' heads to heal them, drawing it from inside their own chests.

The head soul, it should be noted, is not the seat of consciousness, which is found in the heart soul, also the locus of memory, including the memory of healing songs. If head soul represents vital substance, then, heart soul manifests vital agency. The heart also experiences emotions. Anger, for example, heats and compacts the heart (Roseman 1991, 32) and can lead to illness. The odor of a person's body, particularly in the lower back, is also important. Cutting across someone's personal space can unbind their odor and again cause illness. Finally, there is also a shadow soul, which leaves the body at death. Roseman relates all of these concepts together as "multiple, detachable components of self" (45) but goes on to say that they constitute the Temiar "person" (46). (Self and person are thus brought into relation: selves are multiple, but the person is a unity.) Insightfully, she notes that there is a tension between egocentric and sociocentric components:

> Temiar interactions with one another and the cosmos are driven by a dynamic tension that, on one hand, celebrates the potential detachability of self, and on the other, guards the integrity of self. The cultural subscript of sociocentric interdependence, then, is the continual reinstatement of an independent, bounded self. (47)

With this formulation Roseman advances considerably beyond Occidentalist or Orientalist contrasts. Health may involve the reinstatement of a boundary, a recovery of substance. Or it may involve the passing on of substance in exchanges between people by means of which they guard each other's head souls. But a broken promise or a gift denied, as well as an excessive gift, can all cause illness.

So far in the Temiar materials we see the following: (1) a theory of souls that also provides a theory of trance, song, and healing; (2) a theory of exchange as a means of guarding health; and (3) a theory of personhood that stresses the dialectics of establishing and passing across boundaries.

In the healing process the spirit guide takes over vocalizing power from the medium. "Temiar mediums describe the displacement of their own self while the spirit guide sings through them as 'one's heart is elsewhere'" (Roseman 1991, 115). Besides displacement there is an inversion: the spirit guide comes as a child to the medium, but it is the medium's teacher. The singing draws *kahyek* into the medium and also into his patients, making a cooling force for healing. Mediums are mostly men, but their spirit guides, sometimes seen as their consorts, are often female (here, as in terms of the rest of the data, there is a striking parallel with the Kaluli, Etoro, and others of Papua New Guinea [see Schieffelin 1976; Kelly 1993; Stürzenhofecker 1993]).

Illness results from the transformation of agents inside the body or from the drawing of the head soul out of a patient. The agents come from mountains, fruits, and rivers, and the medium mobilizes the spirit guides from these same sources to combat the agents of illness. The medium is in trance while he heals the patient, and supporters around him also go into trance. The patient need not be in trance. However, since he or she has either lost the head soul or become invaded by the souls of illness agents, it is clear that in Temiar terms a "displacement" has occurred. The displacement is a displacement of the cosmos, its unbinding, and what the medium does is to treat "his patient in the context of a ceremonial performance that reframes reality" (Roseman 1991, 147). The songs do this by referring elaborately to souls of things in the environment itself and bringing their essences to bear on the patient through the creation of sung images. What Roseman calls "disembodied voice" (though that may be an artifact of the embodied-disembodied contrast she uses) becomes transformed into embodied *kahyek*, healing substance.

The healing songs are also a kind of history. As Roseman expresses it: "a vibrant, continuous yet constantly reconstructed history of a people's relationship to their surroundings is encoded in the landscape" (1991, 59). Furthermore, through singing "places become persons, landforms become specific locations" (79). More accurately, perhaps, in the Temiar worldview places and persons both have souls and can interact by means of soul substance.

The Temiar case also shows us that the songs of spirit mediums encode a history and thus constitute a mode of historical consciousness and that healing is the invocation of that consciousness as a means of reframing the patient's experience. Whether the patient is in trance or not, the experience created is one that is entranced and rests on a heightened sense of embodied knowledge/practice concentrated in singing. From a cultural or sociogenic view the key term here is the cosmos; from a psychogenic view it is that of reframing experience within the cosmos. Clearly, there is no contradiction between these views.

Wana Shamanship: Opening Hidden Realms

The Wana people of Sulawesi in Indonesia practice *mabolong*, a shamanic healing ritual in which drumming and singing play central parts. Shamans summon spirit familiars as Temiar mediums do spirit guides: there is more emphasis, however, on the power of the shaman to attract the familiar to him. The shaman's songs also define a local sense of community as well as encapsulating references to past history.

They depend on a division of the world into the visible and the invisible, or hidden: only shamans know how to enter the invisible realm. This realm is also the realm of the glorious past, the source of power. When the shaman invokes it, his "summons has the potential to be at once nostalgic and powerful: nostalgic because of its multiple allusions to past shamans and to an era of magic, powerful because the shaman conjures a potent concentration of hidden being around him" (Atkinson 1989, 76). At healing sessions, either with the full dramatics of the *mabolong* or simply as *potudu* (private healing encounters), the shaman begins by summoning his own powerful familiar to help him with the diagnosis of an illness and either to extract an object from the patient's body or to recover a part of the patient's being (soul): for example, the body soul in the back, the dream agent, and the pulse points in the hands and feet (86). By invoking his familiar, the shaman can augment his own vision with theirs and so perceive the hidden dimensions of existence in a manner the Wana compare to dreaming and that Atkinson suggests we might gloss as an altered state of consciousness (92). One shaman explained to Atkinson that when he closed his eyes he saw visions and when he opened them his thoughts snapped back without an elaborate transition. During his visions the shaman is also aware of his (ordinary) thoughts and feelings (93). This description is consistent with a state of light, self-induced trance.

Shamans are potentially ambiguous figures. They may control spirit familiars who are in fact liver-eating demons or vampires that possess X-ray vision. By implication they might use them to do harm. The shaman also in his *mabolong* performances may "assume the personalities and desires of his spirit allies" (Atkinson 1989, 99), and, if audience members do not indulge the spirits with their requests for special foods or other presents, the shaman's soul may go off with the spirit in a huff. In this regard, although we cannot perhaps speak of full-blown spirit possession, it is evident that the shaman may be a host to spirits whose personalities fuse with his own through the *mabolong*.

The context of ideas about personhood within which shamanism operates is important. *Koro* refers to the living body, also to "a soullike component of self" that resides in a person's upper back but may be absent in illness and survives death (Atkinson 1989, 104). *Tanuana* is the dream self, which can also be startled out of the body, again resulting in illness. Liver (*ate*), scalp skin (*pela mwo'o*) and brains (*uta*) are vital elements that may be stolen from the body and recovered by a shaman.

In sum "the person . . . is a fragile concatenation of hidden elements that are prone to disperse of their own accord or at the will of external agents" (114). Wana perceive a homology between person in this sense and polity and see shamans as both healing persons and holding the community together (118). *Mabolong* performances are as significant for the spectators in general as for the sick person, and Atkinson notes that the role of the actual patient "is passive and usually minor" (124). The patient does not engage in dialogue with the healer and shows no signs of entering trance. Neither hypnotism nor applied psychotherapy are at work. Atkinson briefly considered the problem of therapeutic efficacy and the effect of healing on the patient. She notes that the patients may not hear the words of the shaman's song but probably knows them anyway and that the patient, like the spectators, is further drawn into the healing context through music and dance.

The second half of Atkinson's book is in fact concerned with the shaman's community role, and she compares shamans to the role type posited for New Guinea by Maurice Godelier of the "great man," since shamans, unlike Melanesian big men, do not have direct control over production but, rather, over mystical power (Godelier and Strathern 1991). The shaman acts as a centripetal force in a small community through exercise of influence and by invoking spirits of mythology and of the periphery. He creates an embryonic history based on a myth of nostalgia for a "great" past in which power was putatively more centralized. The Wana shaman therefore defines a modal historical consciousness that we can see as intermediate between that of the Temiar and of the Trengganu people of Malaysia, whom I consider next.

In therapeutic terms the Wana case closely resembles the Temiar: psychogenic and sociogenic components mesh through the concept of the cosmos. Shamans are managers of modal states of consciousness, and Wana historical consciousness is rather more expansive than that of the Temiar, while it supports a nostalgia for the past that is, in fact, only a backdrop to the shaman's contemporary claims to influence.

The Trengganu: "Unusual Illness" and Inner Winds

Atkinson points out that Wana magic has borrowed casually from Islamic traditions. Laderman's study of the Trengganu of Malaysia shows a much stronger overlay of Islamic humoral ideas on indigenous practices. The *bomoh*, or traditional healers, she studied were somewhat under attack from the authorities of the Islamic state religion; in fact, their practices may have been modified in deference to Islamic law.

Nevertheless certain aspects of Trengganu healing appear distinctive from either Islamic notions or the two cases sketched earlier. Most notably there is an emphasis on "inner winds" (angin) that are present at birth and "will determine the child's individual personality, drives, and talents" (Laderman 1991, 41). Inner winds are related to the Breath of Life and the Spirit of Life, Semangat. This spirit can easily be startled (like the Temiar head soul). Some people's boundaries are said to be "riddled with tiny openings," and their thoughts easily become confused. Bomoh shamans call on their familiars to guard these boundaries and strengthen them. Those they invoke are "the Four Sultans, the Four Heroes, the Four Guardians, and the Four Nobles" (43). These are clearly mythologically/historically conceived of spirits, and they may be conjured up by the bomoh in the same way as the Wana shaman calls on his familiar. The patient's thoughts, however, must also be in harmony with those of the bomoh; otherwise, healing will not work.

The bomoh is visited by an array of spirits, one of whom reveals the cause of the patient's illness. The bomoh exorcises the guilty spirit that has brought the illness about and the patient goes into trance and is encouraged to dance. The patient, however, is not thought of as directly possessed; rather, he or she is affected by angin, a forceful wind internal to his or her own body. The shaman also is not strictly possessed but, instead, senses the spirits in his trance state. His own familiar spirits prevent the hostile spirits from entering his body (Laderman 1991, 61).

The term angin can mean simply wind, or chill, in the humoral sense. But it can also refer to individual or capricious desires or to sadness in the liver. Inner winds are like the person's temperament, which makes the person apt for a particular way of life. If the angin is thwarted, sickness can result. Iconic versions of personality types are represented in folklore, and, when a patient is in trance, he or she will rise and dance out the archetypal character to which his or her angin corresponds. Laderman, clearly interested in therapeutic efficacy and in psychogenic theories, compares the Trengganu theory to the ideas of Freud and Jung, concluding that there is a parallel in terms of the idea of blocked creativity. She notes, however, that, whereas psychiatrists discuss mental disorders as examples of "neurosis," Malay shamans do not, nor do they think of angin as developing (like "the self" in western thought) out of social experiences; instead it is there from birth (Laderman 1991, 79). Cautiously, she accepts a parallel between *angin* and Jungian archetypes (80). She argues that shamans bring *angin* to consciousness through trance in the same way as Jungian psychologists bring archetypes into the open. We see here an analogy turning into a translation turning into a generalization of a psychogenic kind, since she argues that "this is an important part of the work of the Malay shamans" (81).

Laderman offers a number of scenarios that may contribute to the further understanding of healing in Trengganu. Spirit divination can locate the cause of illness outside of the patient and thus preclude blame and conduce toward recovery. The divination may work once and for all or may have to be repeated—for example, if a divorced man is plagued by his ex-wife's spirit (Laderman 1991, 82). But sufferers from *angin* have to accept that their sickness is internally caused and express their emotions (e.g., rage) in trance (the permission to do so enables catharsis). Laderman quotes Finkler's reference to Kiev's work, which regards "autonomous individuality" as central to Western psychiatry, though it is absent in the Mexican spiritualist healing studied in detail by Finkler (83). Contrary to the usual accounts of Southeast Asian (or for that matter Melanesian, we may add) concepts, Laderman argues that in the Malay case the idea of "individual susceptibility" is central (but the question of "autonomy" is perhaps a separate one). Finally, Laderman notes that, for therapy to work, healer and patient must to some extent share the same mythology, and she refers to the work of Freud and Jung as mythmaking in this context, making a relativistic twist here in the manner of Catherine Lutz (see Lutz 1985, 1988). And she suggests that her Trengganu materials offer "the sole example in the ethnographic record of an indigenous non-Western method of non-projective psychotherapy existing within the context of a shamanistic seance" (85). If we look outside of shamanism, however, we can find parallels—for example, in the Hagen people's use of the notion of *popokl* anger and the need to confess it if healing is to be achieved (see A. J. Strathern 1968, 1981, 1993a–b; M. Strathern 1968, 1988).

Laderman's study pays much more attention to the patient than does Atkinson's, presumably because of the theory of *angin* that holds in the Malay case. Her extensive renderings of actual séances amply show that the pattern of referring to mythological historical characters found among the Wana is even more elaborated by the Trengganu. Shamans in fact construct whole mythologies and genealogies of the world and invoke the spirits of rajahs and military commanders of the past, partly because rajahs are held to have cool, white blood rather than the hot, red blood of ordinary people (Laderman 1991, 313). One of the winds, white wind, is in fact the title of a rajah. We see here the blending of humoral ideas with concepts of political and ritual hierarchy. The "cool white" blood of the rajahs is also reminiscent of *kahyek* healing fluid blown into the patient's fontanelle by Temiar mediums.

Sociogenically, Malay *bomoh* clearly enact a cosmos and one that is "heavier" with history and the perception of centralized power than is seen in the Wana and a fortiori the Temiar cases. The *bomoh* is not the political focus in his community, but he invokes the aura of centralizing myths of power from history, and these "outside" spirits assist him in healing. He clearly defines a historical consciousness. As clearly also, trancing is significant both for healer and patient, and the patient's agency is expected to be at work in the healing for *angin* sickness, as it is not in the Temiar and Wana instances. Whether this difference is related to historical circumstances is not clear. We can perhaps suggest that a disjunction between personal desires and social circumstances may arise more systematically in contexts in which hierarchy is more marked, a notion that would fit with Bourguignon's original hypothesis linking possession to hierarchy. I am not convinced of any "necessity" in this regard, however. More modestly, we may suggest that trancing does lend special force to the "symbolic reframing of experience" that is an element in all healing rituals, and it is therefore especially appropriate to conditions in which such reframing is considerable and faces difficulties.

Atkinson has recently discussed and compared her own work with that of Laderman in an article surveying the continuity and expansion of shamanistic practices generally. She points out that changes in attitude to the phenomenon of shamanism have resulted from new understandings of the term *altered states of consciousness*, or *ASC*, though anthropologists have been cautious of accounts that are based on neurophysiology (Atkinson 1992, 311). She herself notes with approval an approach via embodiment. Quoting Gilbert Rouget (1985, 319), who seems himself to have been echoing Marcel Mauss, she writes, "to shamanize is as much a corporeal technique as a spiritual exercise" (Atkinson 1992, 312). She takes up also the question of shamanism as therapy, noting that it has "been explained in terms of everything from metaphors to endorphins" (313). She cites the "experiential mosaics" invoked by Robert Desjarlais in his study of the embodied aesthetics of Nepalese shamans and the "transfer of secreted opioid peptides" by Kung dancers to patients whom they rub with sweat (Desjarlais 1989, 1992; Frecska 1989). Atkinson accepts the possibility of these and other factors being at work and agrees with Laderman's argument that Malaysian shamanistic therapy should be considered as on a level with Western (e.g., Jungian) psychotherapy. She does note, though, that shamanic performances may be concerned with other issues rather than, or besides, healing, and in particular she restates cross-culturally the connection between shamanism and politics that she found among the Wana (315). (See also A. J. Strathern 1994a, on some Melanesian cases.)

Atkinson also points out that psychological and sociological approaches to healing and shamanism are usually contrasted, but she advocates, as I do here, that we should try to bring them together under the rubric of ethnopsychologies. I continue my own efforts in this direction by shifting now to Madagascar and thence to mainland Africa, beginning with the Mayotte people studied by Michael Lambek.

The Mayotte: Embodiment and Objectification

In two separate works Michael Lambek (1981, 1993) has elaborated an impressive cultural account of trance among the Mayotte people that builds successively on metaphors of "text" and "embodiment." In both monographs the focus is on the cultural construction of knowledge and the practical contexts of its deployment. Lambek points out that spirit possession implies an elementary triangle of communication between a spirit, its host, and a third party who must mediate between the first two, an intermediate consciousness that enables two different manifestations located within the same person to speak to each other. Implicit here is the idea that the host does not consciously hear what the spirit says and therefore cannot "remember" what happens during the period of possession. We would have to argue, then, that possession involves deep trance (unless we are to assume that everything is the result of intentional role playing). Extrapolating a little, we can argue that possession intrinsically involves either blockage or contradiction or both and is itself a way of transcending contradiction. I do not mean this proposition to be taken in a straightforward functionalist sense but, rather, that it is part of a general model of the communicative process in possession—also, as I will argue, that it is symptomatic of certain kinds of history.

In his latest work Lambek concentrates on experts who have learned to accommodate and manage a number of spirits, who impart to him or her their knowledge. Modifying the metaphor of text he used in the earlier work, he writes:

> Possession is constituted by a practice and politics of voice rather than of text, of speaking rather than reading, of body rather than of intellect. . . . By its very nature possession finds the source of its authority in the embodiment of knowledge. A medium acquires and lays claim to knowledge by the public fact and personal experience of trance and by the coherence of his or her performance. (Lambek 1993, 306).

Embodiment is what makes the knowledge experientially real; its producer, however, has to objectify it in the personage of the spirit. There is, therefore, a dialectic of objectification and embodiment. Here Lambek directly follows Bourdieu, who applied his insight to the use of the body in culturally encoded space (Bourdieu 1977, 87). It was an important insight and led directly to the ascendance of the concept of embodiment in anthropological writing in the 1980s. Lambek also draws inspiration from Fortes's work on taboo, since taboos are embodied rules, transcending the gap between language and act. On these insights Lambek builds his own detailed and sympathetic picture of how a medium gradually builds up a coherent personality for the spirit who possesses him or her and uses this in practical life. The communicative function is in prime focus, and the context is sociogenic. Some questions of consciousness, however, remain.

If the host is in deep trance and does not remember what happens when possession takes place, how can the personality of the spirit be built up? Only through the mediation of others, whose consciousness therefore enters into the construction. This may help to explain how spirits become socially relevant. But in another sense it is possible to discern that by cultivating a range of spirits a medium actually acquires a level of individuation that would otherwise be denied. Through the spirits he or she can reveal aspects and desires that otherwise could not appear. Classic cases of this phenomenon are well-known in the *Zar* cults of North Africa, but the Mayotte case shows the same structural potentiality. Furthermore, we may suggest that the "oppositional" character of possession is everywhere heightened as a result of the spread of Islam and the diffusion of gender ideology that goes with it. It is here that the question of historical consciousness also reenters. (It is also important to note, in passing, that possession cults *themselves* are subject to processes of diffusion [see Lewis n.d.]).

At Lombeni, where Lambek worked, two kinds of spirits were held to possess people, the *trumba* and the *patros* (Lambek 1993, 310). Patros spirits are usually male and belong to a general type shared between the Near East and both East and West Africa. Senior *trumba* spirits represent deceased royal rulers of the Sakalava states of northwestern Madagascar. Younger *trumba* represent nineteenth-century social classes—e.g., warriors, sailors, slaves. They are not village ancestors. It is apparent that these spirits encode and are the sole current manifestation of a complex and partly pre-Islamic history. They are "contradictory" to the present, since they belong unambiguously to the past, and a powerful past at that (in a manner reminiscent of the way Wana spirits are regarded by their shamans). In brief, I suggest that the contradictory character of these spirits, and their powerful aura, fits well with the contradictory way in which they stand for aspects of individuation that set possessed persons at odds with some aspects of their defined social roles. If this is correct, the overall form of "consciousness" that is at work is one that operates at two levels: historical/social and individual/psychic. Again, a homology between sociogenic and psychogenic components is found. That the one merges into the other can also be seen in the interesting fact that a child may take on its parent's spirits, in competition with and eventually replacement of the elder generation: another locus for the dialectic of objectification and embodiment (see Lambek 1993, 324).

In his later work Lambek is not so much concerned with the question of illness. Possession, however, is seen initially as a kind of illness, and cultivating the spirits is a kind of therapy. When it is recognized that a spirit is rising to the head of a patient, a curer puts the patient into trance, listens to the demands of the spirit, and negotiates with it (Lambek 1981, 47). The curer is also one who has spirits who help him in extracting sorcery objects and in diagnosing illness generally. The curer relays the spirit's demands to the host. Feasts are held to placate the spirit until the host is able to have a stable relationship with it. The crucial point here is that the patient is first *put* into trance by a curer and then later learns to *manage* his or her trance: thus, there is an achievement of consciousness in control over trancing, a feature shared everywhere by mediums and shamans. Indeed, when we look at the phenomenon of possession, as opposed to trance without possession, it is clear that possession is frequently signaled by, or interpreted as a form of illness (and vice versa) and that the cure for it is *not* exorcism, necessarily, but acceptance of an ongoing relationship (called by some anthropologists "advocism" [Lewis n.d.]). Such a perspective strengthens the idea that it represents a development of the consciousness of the host, even though a formal separation between host and spirit is maintained based on the assertion of noncommunication, that is, on the ethnomodel of deep trance. It is equally evident that this separation is maintained by the position that the spirits involved are figures from the historical past. This latter point can be made even more clearly from the next case, that of the Songhay.

Fusion of Worlds, Fission of the Person: The Songhay

Paul Stoller has given us a deeply felt study of Songhay possession in his book *Fusion of the Worlds* (1989a). The Songhay people of Niger in West Africa have a long and complicated history, centered around the founding and dissolution of local dynasties of rulers and their tributary relations to other kingdoms, for example, in Ghana and Mali. The Songhay themselves established an empire that flourished from 1493 to 1591 and then declined through internecine rivalries. They remained a stratified patrilineal society with a strong distinction between nobles and slaves and a subordinate status for women generally. Finally, they were conquered by the French colonial army at the end of the nineteenth century. From the sixteenth century onward they were also much influenced by Islam.

An equally complicated set of spirits can be involved in possessing mediums and their patients. For example, the Tooru spirits date back to the time of empire in the early sixteenth century; Genji Kawri spirits, from the same era, represent Islamic incursions; the Genji Bi represent indigenous peoples conquered by the Songhay; Hausa spirits reflect mercantile influences of the early twentieth century; and the Hauka are from French colonial times. "Each spirit family, then, signifies a distinct historical period during which there occurred a sociocultural crisis"

(Stoller 1989a, 30). The Songhay case, therefore, offers a perfect example of tendencies observed in preceding instances: the preservation and representation of historical forces in the realm of spirit possession and the relationship of possession not simply with hierarchy but also with historical rupture and contradiction—"crisis" in Stoller's succinct term (see also Kapferer 1992).

There is a pervasive theme, therefore, of the appropriation of power from the past and in a sense from the "outside." In a manner reminiscent of Mary Douglas's formulations danger comes from the outside. But danger is also power, available to be socialized. The body as the medium for such power has also to be conceptualized as a mindful, intentional body, even though the prime image of possession makes of the host's body something apparently passive. According to Adamu Jenitongo, a Songhay seer and medium, the human body consists of flesh, life force, and the double (bia). Life force is in the heart, and it leaves at death. Spirit mediumship results from the displacement not of life force but of the double. The spirit is an invisible double that becomes visible in the host's body by displacing the host's double temporarily. As in the case of the Mayotte, a person who wishes to become a medium must come to terms with the possessing spirit. A zima's (medium) children may become possessed by his spirits, continuing a line of succession. Possession mediums must separate themselves from Islamic clerics, and to do so they wear black instead of white, noting that "one foot cannot follow two paths" (Stoller 1989a, 37). Zima, therefore, stand generally for indigenous Songhay values as against Islam. Although their activities cannot simply be classified as "resistance," they do show an unmistakable oppositional character. Access to spirits of the past through trance possession enables zima to validate their claims in the face of an Islamic hegemony. Their patients thus participate in the same "oppositional scenario" (a phrase I borrow from Schieffelin [1976], applying it to a different context).

Spirit mediumship also offers a contradictory and resistive role to certain gifted women, one of whom, Gusabu, Stoller describes in his chapter 3 (1989a, 45 ff.). Gusabu outlasted several husbands, was strong-willed, and picked out for favor by the spirits by their making her ill with possession sicknesses. Stoller explicitly notes that becoming a medium and/or entry into a possession troupe "is a refuge from a social world in which women are powerless. Women constitute the majority of the spirit mediums" (49). In turn spirit mediums become

those who treat patients for "resistant" illnesses that result from possession by spirits. The patients are initiated into the proper order of
their spirits and are thus cured of their sickness while permanently taking up a relationship with the spirits themselves. As in the Mayotte
case, personal individuation and the regenesis of historical consciousness go hand in hand. The "unconsciousness" of possession transmutes
itself in the communicative triad into the "consciousness" of an embodied role.

The specificity, hierarchy, and depth of historical experiences
expressed in Songhay possession practices stand at the furthest
remove, in this sense, from the Temiar case, with which I began this
survey (for African parallels to the Songhay case, see the intriguing presentations by Fritz Kramer [1993]). Yet in another sense, and in a different modality, Songhay ethnography doubles back onto the Temiar case,
since it is through music, melodic sound, that trancing is induced or
healing encompassed. As Stoller writes:

> Sound is a powerful sensation in Songhay cultural experience. It is
> the only force that can penetrate the body—hence the emotive
> power of music in the world. Just as the sounds of words are
> important in the practice of sorcery and praise-singing in Songhay,
> so the sounds of certain musical instruments are central to Song-
> hay possession ceremonies. These instruments are the monochord
> violin and the calabash drum. (1989a, 111)

The violin "cries" to the people, and its sound is the sound of the ancestors. "We hear the sound and we know that we are on the path of the
ancestors" (pathway as history) (111). Thus, "the violinist is the human
link between social and spirit worlds" (113). And the drum? Adamu
Jenitongo said "that the sound of the drums reminds the dancers, audi-
ences, and spirits of the battlefield heroics of the Songhay past" (118). A
poetics of nostalgia is turned into a poetics of power (see also Stoller
1989b, 101–12).

In addition, two genres, the *Hauka* and the Sasale performances,
show the oppositional contexts of Songhay possession most clearly.
Stoller describes Hauka as horrific comedy. *Hauka* is a Hausa word
meaning craziness. Among the Songhay Hauka performances are
funny, using obscenity as a challenge to colonially privileged characters. Hauka performers "often wore pith helmets and carry swagger

sticks. Sometimes they took the roles of European army generals who spoke to their troops in Pidgin French or Pidgin English. This frivolous burlesque makes impressionable children cringe and seasoned adults laugh" (1989a, 148). The Hauka in fact embodies the kind of parodic appropriation of the other that we often find also in colonial contexts in Melanesia and the wider Pacific region also (Keesing 1992; Thomas 1992).

The Sasale performances also use obscenity, this time specifically in the context of gender relations and in opposition to Islam. Hauka is connected to the rupture of French colonialism, Sasale to modernization in the twentieth century. Sasale prostitute spirits, who outrageously challenge their spectators, "mock the practices of a neoconservative Islam that . . . threatens the very foundation of Songhay society" (Stoller 1989a, 169). Carnivalesque practices thus attempt to invert consciousness, to render ridiculous what has become normative, to show turbulence and negation beneath conformity, to emerge as spirits of protest against the perceived sickness of society.

Elements of this kind lead us easily into the last ethnographic case, the Hofriyati, studied by Janice Boddy.

Hofriyati Homologies: The Enclosure of Women and the Disclosure of Spirits

Janice Boddy's study of the zar cult in the Northern Sudan was intended primarily as a criticism of I. M. Lewis's theory of peripheral possession as protest. She made her case convincingly by encompassing, rather than completely demolishing, Lewis's. By concentrating on women's experience and seeing the cult through their eyes, she was able successfully to show how it had validity from their viewpoint and not simply as a means of opportunistic protest against male domination and lack of care. First incidents of possession illness do sometimes correlate with adverse circumstances in a woman's life cycle: a husband's marriage to another wife, a state of infertility, an event of miscarriage, the death of a child. Spirits tend to follow female links of kinship (Boddy 1989, 242), and their attacks thus stand in contrapuntal relationship with the patrilineal ties stressed by Islam. A woman's body, closed by pharaonic circumcision and opened only for legitimate reproductive activity, comes to stand both for the closed boundaries of village society and for "the cultural over-determination of women's selfhood" (252). A woman can experience her "not-self" only through possession by *zayran* spirits, who are all "alien," from the outside. Boddy explicitly uses the triad of terms *"self, person, individual"* here, arguing a woman is highly socialized into realizing herself as a normative person, but this means she does not achieve individuation. Spirit possession enables her to embrace her experience of otherness while recognizing the spirits "consciously as aspects of her being over which she has limited if potentially increasing control." The latter part of this observation resonates with what we have seen for the Mayotte and the Songhay. Symbolic reframing of experience is also at play, Boddy notes, since, for example, the spirits make infertile a woman who is otherwise fertile (255). She emphasizes that the spirit does not become integrated with the perceived self of the female host. Instead, she writes, "the felt presence of an ever expandable, multiple non-self enhances by opposition a woman's sense of personhood" (256). Later Boddy argues that through possession trance "the culturally determined self may be felicitously repositioned, perhaps transcended.

The experience of trance and its observation in others is the locus of possession's creativity, for in trance a woman becomes, legitimately if temporarily, non-Hofriyati" (Boddy 1989, 350). This formulation corresponds to Hofriyati women's own formulations, since in trance they declare that they see with the eyes of the European or West African spirit that possesses them (in the same way as the Wana shaman sees with the eyes of his spirit allies). Overall, however, a woman does not fuse with her *zayran*. "Human and spirit contextualize each other, maintain each other in contraposition" (353). In general Boddy sees possession and its curing as a means whereby Hofriyati women come to terms with themselves. Trance is important, because it involves heightened susceptibility to emotional experience, but insight comes perhaps "in remembering her trance experiences" (354; Boddy cites also here Kapferer 1986, 198). This again, I think, is an important point: what people make of trance *consciously* in communication contributes its meanings to the definitions of self and non-self that go with it. Boddy's analysis here heads in the same direction as Lambek has taken in his later work on the Mayotte.

Who, then, are these alien spirits that are pulled into a social dialectic with the Hofriyati women's world? The Hofriyati have been frequently invaded by several peoples over the last four thousand years: ancient Egyptian, Meroitic Christian, Arabic, Mameluke, Funj, and Turkish, and British. They are a people who have been overrun many times, whose boundaries have always been transgressed, and whose menfolk have most recently been drawn into the global political economy through wage labor. Performances by possessed women act as a conduit into fragments of this long history of "dispossession." In one sequence described by Boddy a sick woman was possessed by Westerner spirits; she imitated a military officer in a desert corps conducting a drill and then requested cigarettes, a European belt, a radio, and she flourished a cane. This woman elaborately shook Boddy's hand in "Western" style, threatened to pull a sword, and saluted. Another woman made sweeping flourishes also with a sword; another engaged in formal combat with a transvestite attendant. The next day the sick woman appeared as a lady dressed in green and sprinkled with Evening in Paris cologne. And a further woman was possessed by a Catholic priest, offered benedictions, then also attacked a man with her sword (Boddy 1989, 126 28).

It is impossible not to recognize the elements of licensed reversal, carnival, and parodic appropriation of the other in these vivid portrayals. Hofriyati women are *bricoleurs* of historical consciousness, appropriating as they wish, and these portraits of their non-selves are surely also examples of "individuation" as I have noted for the Mayotte, and of resistive parody, as I have noted for the Songhay Sasale spirits. The conscious, communicative, intentional aspect of possession trance is made apparent, even as the ideology of trance enables both spectators and performers to deny that it is the women themselves who are doing all this. Individuation occurs also through its denial, the putative possession by the other.

Mind-Body Healing, Trance, and the Concept of Embodiment

Trancing seems to play a variable role in the processes of healing exemplified in the cases I have looked at here. There is, for instance, the difference between cases in which the healer enters trance, the patient does so, or both do. Indeed, it is difficult to be precise about the concept of trance itself or to be sure that we are dealing with an altered state of consciousness as against a dramatic performance (not that these two are incompatible). Whatever the context, however, one feature seems to reappear, and that is that healing involves a reframing of experience in the classic manner suggested by James Dow (1986). Trance in turn facilitates such a reframing, as does spirit possession. At one end of the continuum we may be dealing with a new image presented to a patient, at the other with a whole new persona, an alter ego juxtaposed to the self, as in the Hofriyati example. Either a metaphor or a historical figure may be in focus: in either case the result is an altered state of consciousness that whether trance induced or not conduces toward a patient's recovery, a process in which health and identity are brought into consonance with each other. It is important also to recognize that the reframing may involve more than just the individual patient, since spectators are also involved (see Connor 1990).

Ernest Rossi, in collaboration first with Milton Erickson and later with David Cheek, has developed a set of concepts, built into psychotherapeutic practices, that bear on this phenomenon (Erickson 1980; Rossi and Cheek 1988). Their psychotherapeutic work has focused to some extent on the recovery of traumatic memories and hypnosis is used as a means of accessing such memories when suppressed. A novel feature of the approach is the significance given to remarks made by medical personnel and remembered by patients who were in a state of shock, pain, or partial anesthesia when they overheard the remarks. Memory itself is influenced by the state of the brain during an experience, expressible as a configuration of acetylcholine, catecholamine, and serotonin systems. Endocrinal hormones and their peptide analogs "are similarly involved in memory and modulation." From observations such as these Rossi has developed what he calls the "state-dependent memory, learning, and behavior theory of mind-body healing in therapeutic hypnosis." Instead of regarding state-dependent learning as an exotic variant, Rossi proposes it as "the broader, more generic form of learning that takes place in all complex organisms that have a cerebral cortex and limbic-hypothalamic system modulating the expression of Pavlovian and Skinnerian conditioning" (Rossi and Cheek 1988, 109).

Physiological features of the body are also state-dependent and obviously related to health and illness. Rossi has argued that the limbic-hypothalamic and other related systems are the means whereby information is transduced between the brain and the rest of the body (or the mind and the body). Accordingly, all methods of mind-body healing must operate by "accessing and reframing the state-dependent memory and learning systems that encode symptoms and problems" (Rossi 1986, 55; qtd. in Rossi and Cheek 1988, 111).

Rossi has also advanced some remarks on the relationship of learning to consciousness. In early selection theory, as proposed by Broadbent, "consciousness is primary and necessary for memory and learning." In this mode the person actively selects from the flow of experience what to remember and discards the rest. In late selection theory, however, which Rossi espouses, "consciousness is secondary and not necessary for memory and learning," even, for example, for "highly skilled neurological and perceptual activities which include language understanding" (Rossi and Cheek 1988, 15).

These remarks can be brought to bear on trancing, as Rossi and Cheek intend. Trancing, whether through hypnosis or not, may enable a patient to recover memories encoded without conscious attention. Equally, it may enable new learning and new memories to be established. In trance, if any early selection against certain kinds of information is ordinarily practiced, such a tendency is neutralized. The patient is in a state of high receptivity. Exactly the same applies to the case in which it is the shaman, not the patient, who is in trance. But in the ethnographic cases we have considered the process of learning and reframing is not *confined* to trance episodes. What is revealed in trance is assimilated in other contexts, and the holistic nature of experience is facilitated by the fact, according to Rossi and Cheek, that "many of the sensory-perceptual languages of the mind . . . are encoded like a map over the cortex . . . [and] . . . can be transduced or transformed into one another via the 'cross-modal association areas' of the limbic system." They go on to suggest, in fact, that such transduction can be termed "consciousness." "Consciousness [is] a process of self-reflective information transduction" (Rossi and Cheek 1988, 162). In other words it can be seen as a means of reflecting on state-dependent learning. Finally, such within-brain processes are closely linked to overall bodily states, since "certain neurons within the hypothalamus of the brain convert the neural impulses of *mind* into the hormonal *information substances* of the body" (163). Such a model, they point out, can be used, for example, to update Hans Selye's theory of stress as transmitted by the autonomic, endocrine, and immune systems, since "the limbic-hypothalamic-pituitary system of the brain plays the major integrative role in the mind modulation of all three of these major systems" (164). The process of information transduction continues down via receptors to the cellular level.

As Rossi and Cheek recognize, "the current challenge is to determine just how and where hypnosis enters these cybernetic loops to facilitate mind-body healing" (1988, 167). Although hypnosis is a special case, we could also substitute *trance* for *hypnosis* in this formulation. Overall, however, this sketch of information transduction indicates that (1) there can be a complex translation from mental images into cellular modifications and (2) consciousness plays a major role in facilitating such patterns. Such indications fall into line with the evidence of the communicative processes that surround trance and healing in the ethnographic cases I have examined. For these cases, however, we have also to extend the domain of consciousness further, since we have seen a consistent pattern in societies with complex histories for aspects of these histories to be encoded in possession trance behavior. It is as though the state-dependent theory of learning and memory had here been written large on the canvas of social history. Possession memory culturally encodes historical "state-dependent" experiences, bringing these back also into alignment with individual experiences in a sliding scale. Such a work of "analogous memory" has to be seen both as a creative act of consciousness and a recovery of suppressed and therefore unconscious experience.

Rossi's work significantly collapses the mind-body dichotomy, although it does give much primacy to brain-centered experience. Given this, what becomes of the concept of embodiment? Like many others we have used in anthropology, it too can now be relativized. Matters acted out through the body as embodied knowledge are also linked with brain transduction processes. Quite differently, ethnographic cases also show the relativity of the concept, since mind-body concepts themselves vary cross-culturally. Is the head soul of the Temiar a part of the Temiar "body" or not, for example? In Songhay spirit possession the spirit double replaces the human double: Is it a part of the body or not? At least the concept of embodiment, like that of the body, is problematized, along with concepts such as "symbolic or metaphorical action."

Just as Paul Stoller has insisted on a "fusion of the worlds" in his study of Songhay possession (1989), so we may insist on a fusion of mind and body and of consciousness and unconsciousness in the kinds of expressions healers have invented in different cultures to achieve the reframing of experience. I know of no better example of this than one given by Kaja Finkler in her study of spiritualist healing in Mexico, in which she writes of Chucha, a female patient with chronic problems of chest pain who was told by her healer that her heart palpitations should be thought of as "crystalline drops falling into an empty glass, the drops symbolizing God's words transmitted during irradiations [spiritualist church services] and Chucha representing the empty glass" (1985, 171–72). In this image, with its transposition, or information transduction, from the body to the word via an extrasomatic comparison, we see exemplified the general form of what from our perspective we call "symbolic healing." Often connected with the potential of such images to calm the patient and aided by a mild condition of trance in which "cortical excitation is diminished," the ergotropic system is less active, and the trophotropic system of the body is stimulated (164).

The idea of cortical encoding with information transduction between different sites in the brain facilitated through the limbic system fits well enough with anthropological theories of the power of symbols and their "cognitive" and "visceral" poles, as Victor Turner put it. As an example, we can cite here Robert Desjarlais's recent work on body aesthetics and healing in Nepal. Desjarlais argues that we must recognize the existence of unique grammars of experience seen in embodied aesthetics of experience (1992, 62). His particular argument is that such aesthetics are not the recondite province of shamans but, rather, must be shared widely by the populace at large in everyday life. Desjarlais insists also that aesthetics pervade many dimensions of life, not only those labeled as "artistic." He mounts an intricate discussion on the links between physiological and social processes, using ideas from both Gregory Bateson and Pierre Bourdieu to complement each other. He refers here to "somatic sensibilities" of the Yolmo people whom he studied, which are equally physiological, cultural, and at times political, and he usefully reminds us that in these matters it is not only meaning that is at stake but also values.

Indeed, this is the vital link to make in terms of the crossover between the physiological and the political. Value is given to the physiological by the political (and perhaps vice versa). Desjarlais develops a Yolmo poetics of the concrete by moving, as he says, from tangible image to felt quality (Desjarlais 1992, 71). Embodied experience is thus the touchstone of his exposition. "A phenomenology of Yolmo aesthetics," he writes, "must begin and end with the body. . . . And since aes-

thetic (and hence moral and political) values emanate from, and take
root within, the body, we return to the realm of the sensory." He goes
on to outline the dimensions of Yolmo aesthetics that have to do with
"harmony, control, integration, presence, and purity" (70) and links
these to micropolitical processes within the village (as Atkinson does
for the Wana people). Yolmo aesthetics turn out to be akin to classic
humoral theories of the body/group, with their emphasis on balance
and harmony of forces among people, who are themselves seen as the
"bearers of organic mosaics" (74). This image of the mosaic or network
of associations that makes up the embodied person is quite consistent
with Rossi and Cheek's concept of information transduction, and
through it we can build a shared set of meanings for the work *embodiment,* since cultural embodiments may be enacted or coded within the
brain itself. In any case, we meet here again the prominence of the term
embodiment, to which I will now turn, after this examination of ethnotheories of trance and healing and their possible counterparts in the
state-dependent theory of learning.

Chapter 8

Embodiment

The problems of analyzing trance and possession in relation to cross-cultural healing practices have brought us face to face again with questions of mind-body relations, of consciousness, and of the embodiment of meaning. Several works produced in the last decade have converged on the importance of this concept of embodiment, which also was a focus in chapter 2 of this book, as reflected in the ideas of Pierre Bourdieu and Paul Connerton on habitus and memory. Embodiment, however, as it has been deployed by a range of theorists, has come to have a fan of referents that takes it further than being synonymous with Bourdieu's habitus concept. In this chapter I will look at a set of writings that have contributed to this process of enrichment of meaning of the term and have argued that it is central in today's anthropology. I consider first Thomas Csordas's 1988 Stirling Award essay in psychological anthropology, which explicitly proposes "embodiment as a paradigm for anthropology" (1990, 5).

Embodiment as Paradigm: Pentecostal Practices

The claim of paradigmatic status here seems grand, yet Csordas's actual aim is quite modest: he offers embodiment as a concept "that encourages reanalyses of existing data and suggests new questions for empirical research" (1990, 5). With this remark he deflects possible suspicion that embodiment is suddenly to be raised to the level of a meta-narrative in the wake of fallen shibboleths from the past. He goes on to explain the affinity between his perspectives and those of phenomenology—in particular, we might say, the work of Merleau-Ponty. With this background he announces that the body is not an object that takes on cultural form but is, in fact, the subject of culture, its "existential ground," in a way similar to Irving Hallowell's concept of "the self." The body is involved in both perception and in practice and therefore

enables us to transcend the duality of subject and object, which Marcel
Mauss had earlier preserved in writing quite separately about "the
techniques of the body" as against "the notion of the person."

As Csordas notes, in order to collapse the dualities of percep-
tion/practice or structure/practice, the body itself has to be a unitary
concept, not opposed to a principle of mind (Csordas 1990, 8). In other
words, the body is the mindful body that has been our constant focus in
this book. It must be noted here that creating a unity in this way does
not obliterate questions and problems to do with mind by referring to
everything as "body" and slipping *mind* back in within the concept of
"embodiment." Rather, we have to think of a mind-body totality operating in the environment in the figure-background manner suggested
by gestalt theorists.

Merleau-Ponty's approach is relativist and stresses the indeterminacy of perception between subject and object (similar to Heisenberg's
uncertainty principle). We would describe this position nowadays as
anticognitivist. Objects do not exist in any a priori sense but only a pos-
teriori, as a result of perception. Hence, objects are the end products of
perception, and perception is always embodied. Merleau-Ponty wants
to capture the beginnings of perception in this sense, starting with what
he calls the "pre-objective" and considering it in opposition to
Durkheim's injunction that we treat social facts as "things." The pre-
objective is not precultural, however; it is simply pre-abstract, corresponding to everyday modes of behavior, which can be specified in
bodily terms.

Csordas brings into alignment Merleau-Ponty's idea of the pre-
objective in perception and Bourdieu's concept of habitus in practice.
These concepts belong together, in the same order of ideas. Bourdieu's
habitus encompasses both mental and somatic functions and thus acts
as a universal mediator explaining how practices come about. Csordas
sees a theoretical contradiction between Merleau-Ponty's phenomenology and Bourdieu's "dialectical structuralism" (although he does not
elaborate what this contradiction is, it must have to do with the definition of "the subject") but notes that, as methodological concepts, their
ideas may be used together, and he proceeds to do so with reference to
his own field studies of Pentecostalism in North America. He takes first
the casting out of evil spirits.

Such spirits are seen by Pentecostals in the medieval mode of
demons that transgress body boundaries and cause "possession." He

makes a useful processual differentiation here between laypersons and healers (priests). In the pre-objective mode (i.e., in immediate experience) persons feel something out of their control in their behavior. The healer then objectifies this pre-objective perception as a case of demonic intrusion. If this distinction is general, it offers us a general model of specialist healing corresponding in biomedicine to the distinction between illness and disease. Commonalities within the pre-objective experience are to be attributed to Bourdieu's habitus. Healing depends on the habitus here, since it rests on the bodily image of expelling the evil spirit—more particularly, on the idea of releasing the victim from control by the spirit so as to reenter into harmony with the spirit of God (consider the Pentecostal chorus "I'm free, I'm free, I'm free to be a servant of the Lord"). In stressing the pre-objective perception of bondage rather than the objective notion of transgression, Csordas argues that he has approached closer to the phenomenological context; that is, he is able to write a more sensitive ethnographic account. Embodiment as such, he says, might lead us either to the pre-objective or to the objective levels. Commenting further, I would say that either level can provide insight: furthermore, in many cultures "transgression" *is* a pre-objective concept. What is pre-objective in one cultural context becomes objectified in another. Such matters, also, as the diagnostic "signature" of an evil spirit depend very much again on habitus (i.e., embodied culture).

Csordas now compares Pentecostal practices with those of Charismatic Catholics. Among these there is also faith healing, indexed by a variety of "signs and wonders" and there is trancelike behavior marked by enhanced bodily sensations that sweep through a congregation (social effervescence) and culminate in "resting in the Spirit," a semi-swooning position, and the revelation of a "word of knowledge." The word of knowledge is the good inverse of incursion by evil spirits in the Pentecostal scheme of things. Somatic images are inculcated: participants are expected to feel heat and heaviness in their bodies and to laugh, cry, or fall as they are affected by the sacred force. Healers are further inspired simply to diagnose conditions (with the risk that they may be wrong). One dominant image is that of water breaking through boundaries and/or cleansing the person from sin or illness. The pre-objective is involved here because the participants' acceptance of diagnoses depends on the habitus, causing them, Csordas says, to misrecognize their source as God rather than the socially informed body itself

(1990, 23). From this he returns to his initial assertion that the lived body is the existential ground of culture (including the sacred). (See also the fuller account in Csordas 1994a.) This existential ground is to be found in the pre-objective—but it must be noted that, while it is the ground of culture, it also already includes culture, since for Merleau-Ponty, as for other phenomenologists, being is already "being in the world," and "the world" is culturally constituted. Although he speaks of an "existential ground," then, Csordas is using a cyclical rather than a linear form of reasoning here.

Csordas's third exemplification of embodiment theory has to do with trance and glossolalia. Glossolalia reveals, as it were, the root of speech, since this, according to Merleau-Ponty, lies in "a verbal gesture with immanent meaning" (Csordas 1990, 25). Glossolalia "reveals language as incarnate," like the Word made Flesh, and Csordas argues that it "takes place at a phenomenological moment prior to distinction between body and mind" (26). The pre-objective is once more brought into focus here.

Finally, Csordas is also able to introduce a historical element into his analysis, since among Charismatic Catholics speaking with tongues corresponded to an initial phase of revival in the 1960s and resting in the spirit came later with a more quietist emphasis in the 1980s. The example indicates clearly how habitus may change over time.

In keeping with Merleau-Ponty's formulations, Csordas's arguments operate continuously within the framework of "culture." He notes, for example, that physiological theories may provide accounts of the mechanisms of trance or of catharsis but cannot explain how these are molded into cultural expressions. His argument here resonates with my own in chapter 7, in which I show that the healing discourses of shamans and/or possessed persons coincide with specific varieties of historical consciousness. Csordas further takes Durkheim to task for declaring "society" to be the force that defines religious power. Csordas seeks this, instead, in embodied experience, as when a thought suddenly occurs to a person or there is an experience of being controlled by another force. Religion thus becomes a particular hermeneutic of experience. And he suggests, finally, that the idea of embodiment may help us to reconcile the distinction between cognition and emotion, asking how thought is embodied and how it is related to affect (Csordas 1990, 37). He ends, therefore, with some large questions that have been broached also both by cognitive scientists and by theorists following in the steps of Silvan Tomkins (1960). And he hazards the metasuggestion that Merleau-Ponty's principle of indeterminacy fits with the shift in postmodernist anthropology from "key symbols to blurred genres" (Csordas 1990, 43). Here it must be noted, however, that he himself relies much more on the identification of key symbols than on blurring of genres. Most useful, overall, is his identification of pre-objective embodied elements in the religious behavior he discusses. The power by which the pre-objective is transformed into the objective is an arena that he takes more or less for granted. Yet, in terms of his own definitions, the value of the embodiment concept for paradigmatic issues is fully demonstrated. Other theorists have tended to look more at the "objectified" end of the scale, as Bourdieu does, although Bourdieu also clearly identifies a dialectic as operating between objectification and embodiment (see also chap. 7, on the Mayotte).

Embodiment is a term that collapses the duality of mind and body, then, essentially by infusing body with mind. Mark Johnson has expressed the reverse part of this process with his image of the body in the mind (1987). I turn next to a consideration of his work along with that of Varela, Thompson, and Rosch in *The Embodied Mind* (Varela et al. 1991).

"Body" and "Metaphor": A Basic Conjunction

Johnson's main aim is to counter what he calls the dominant objectivist theory of meaning and rationality in European philosophy and to replace it with a nonobjectivist theory that includes both embodiment and imagination. Objectivist theory supposes that linguistic meaning is predicated on conditions of satisfaction of the truth of utterances with respect to the real world. Meaning resides in the correspondence between words and things or the correct and neutral labeling of discrete objects by means of discrete linguistic units. In such a theory it is clear that meaning can properly only be literal meaning, and the aim of science would be to reduce all descriptions to such a literal level. Metaphor, therefore, and with it imagination, becomes secondary and is not a serious object of investigation or a fundamental way of conceptualizing the world.

Johnson notes that such objectivist viewpoints have a long philosophical history, stretching back to interpretations of the work of Plato and his rejection of the validity of poetic statements on the grounds that they can reveal only "appearances," not "truth." He singles out Immanuel Kant, however, as a philosopher who seriously attempted to consider the role of imagination in reasoning and who suggested that it is our means of moving from innate categories of the mind (concepts) to sensations (percepts). Knowledge for Kant depended on both sensibility (perception) and understanding (the application of concepts). Imagination was the bridge between them, with a foot in both, as it were (Johnson 1987, 166), but it was not clear how this could be. Johnson argues that the problem here was created by the metaphysical split itself between the formal and the material (corresponding to the mind and the body). This split entails a "rigid separation of understanding from sensation and imagination [which] relegates the latter to second-class status as falling outside the realm of knowledge" (167). If, instead, we abolish this rigid split, imagination can be given an honorable place in the process of reasoning. Kant almost reached this conclusion, Johnson suggests, but drew back. Instead, he ended by reinforcing the gap between reason and bodily experience.

Against this conclusion Johnson invites us to consider that imagination has a constitutive place in embodied reasoning. Understanding, he argues,

> is the way we *"have a world," the way we experience our world as a comprehensible reality.* Such understanding, therefore, involves *our whole being*—our bodily capacities and skills, our values, our moods and attitudes, our entire cultural tradition. . . . In short, our understanding is our "mode of being in the world." (Johnson 1987, 102)

The specific idea that Johnson brings to bear on his argument is his theory of image schemata. Such schemata do not have the rich particularity of a specific mental image; rather, they are like the structural forms that underlie many such images. Working essentially within English language conventions, he identifies many such schemata and shows how they have a basis in bodily experience. The projection of such schemata into different realms of experience is what he calls "metaphorical projection" (in a moment I will discuss this use of the term). As an example of a schema he instances the notion of balance. He points out that this notion depends intrinsically on bodily experience.

"Balancing is an *activity we learn with our bodies* and not by grasping a set of rules or concepts" (Johnson 1987, 74 ff.). Balance is related to equilibrium in the body, whereby we try to maintain an even state—for example, with respect to heat and cold. Johnson argues that through our bodies we develop "preconceptual gestalt (or schematic) structures that operate in our bodily movements, perceptual acts and orientational awareness" (75). This realm of the "preconceptual" corresponds, in fact, to Merleau-Ponty's "pre-objective." Such schemata can then be elaborated and enter into further realms of consciousness—for example, the realm of argument in which the "weight" of opinion is held to exist on one "side" or the other of a debate. Johnson's point is that by a series of creative acts, which he calls metaphorical, we carry over from one context to another certain basic, and ultimately body-based, schemata.

Why does he call these projections "metaphorical"? Johnson notes that he himself has extended this term to enable it to encompass the operation of image schemata generally. In the objectivist view all metaphors must be reducible to literal statements, and this viewpoint is carried over into "comparison theories," which treat metaphors as elliptical similes, likening, for example, time and money in certain definite respects (although not in others) (Johnson 1987, 67). In another set of views metaphors do not simply reflect such similarities but, in fact, create them (Max Black); in yet another metaphors do not "mean" anything because meaning can only be literal meaning, but they intimate (evoke) nonpropositional matters (Donald Davidson). How this evocation occurs is not made clear. In John Searle's view such metaphors are held to work because of nonpropositional connections in what he calls "the Background" (73). It is precisely this Background that Johnson's own work explicates in terms of his exposition of the pervasiveness of embodied image schemata. The metaphors he uncovers are projections or extensions of such schemata and are "carried over" from one context to the next in this sense. Such metaphors are irreducible. They cannot be further translated into literalities. Here is the only caveat that must be entered for the reader of Johnson's work: in order to understand his concept of metaphor, it is necessary to abandon the very literal-metaphorical contrast on which the term is grounded in objectivist theory as well as in nontechnical writings outside of linguistic theory. Insofar as the term is hard to purge of its objectivist background, it might have been better to utilize another term altogether—for example, *extension*—since the basis for any usage for any image schema is the basic image schema itself.

Johnson's overall approach to the problem of meaning carries with it some powerful advantages and contributes substantially to the significance of the term *embodiment*. First, he abolishes the mind-body distinction, which still inhered in Kant's work and foregrounds the concept of imagination as a basis for rationality (for a further insightful discussion of imagination and also a criticism of Johnson in phenomenological terms, see Csordas 1994, chaps. 5–6). Second, he insists on the bodily basis of many image schemata, thus aligning himself with the phenomenological tradition exemplified by Merleau-Ponty. Third, his work fits well with the perspectives of cultural anthropologists, since his "gestalt structures," or "image schemata," are located within cultural ways of life. Fourth, his approach enables him to analyze historical change in image schemata that illuminate the history of Western science. A good example of this is to be found in his account of how Hans Selye came to develop his theory of stress. In this account it becomes apparent that fundamental image schemata are synonymous with paradigms in the Kuhnian sense.

As a student of internal medicine in Prague in 1925, Selye noticed that patients with various infectious diseases presented a set of common symptoms, which were however, of no interest to his professor, who was intent on discovering specific sets of pathogens. Later in his own research Selye found that such nonspecific but recurrent syndromes were produced in rats by injection of different kinds of damaging substances. Eventually, he came to realize that such symptoms reflected a general tendency by organisms to adapt to damage by stressors; hence, he developed his general theory of stress and of the kind of therapy that could support the body against stressors. Johnson comments that Selye's professor taught his students within the image schema of BODY AS MACHINE, whereas Selye later developed his own theory of the BODY AS HOMEOSTATIC MECHANISM (itself an extension of the basic BALANCE image schema). He points out that data irrelevant in one schema (consigned to an amorphous background) become reconfigured and foregrounded within the other schema (a reversal of figure and background in gestalt terms). This example nicely fits with a Kuhnian viewpoint and gives it a neat exposition, enabling us also to see again the point that there is no such thing as neutral data; all relevant data belong to some theoretical viewpoint that is an objectification of a prior image schema. In this treatment, then, embodiment becomes relevant not only to the pre-objective but also to the objectified realm of experience and plays a fundamental part in the construction of rationality. The same overall effect is achieved by Varela and his colleagues in *The Embodied Mind* (1991), with their concept of "enaction."

Embodiment and Cognition: Enaction

Varela and his colleagues contrast their position with that of cognitivists, cognitive scientists who consider that the aim of their work is to investigate purely mental states and processes in accordance with a kind of Cartesian view of the mind. Cognitivists also consider that such mental processes are universal and are separate from the operation of the emotions. (Their viewpoint thus contrasts sharply both with the "state-dependent memory and learning" theory of Rossi and Cheek [see chap. 7] and with the concepts of people such as the Balinese and the Mount Hageners who link emotions and thought together in a unified notion of the mind and the person.) Recent cognitive science has developed around the idea of the mind as a digital computer. (Johnson would call this an image schema or head metaphor.) Computers of this sort operate on symbols arranged in accordance with a digital code, and this code functions to provide a set of representations of things in the world. By analogy, cognitivists argue, the human mind operates with mental representations that it then proceeds to manipulate in order to produce computations. The mind uncovered by cognitive science thus becomes a "computational mind" and one that succeeds in working with real properties of the world by making internal representations of them. Cognitivism is thus linked to realism in philosophical terms. (For a philosophical-mathematical attack on the idea that consciousness is computational, see Penrose 1994.)

Against this paradigm of cognition Varela and his colleagues suggest that we should use the term *enaction* to emphasize that cognition is "the enactment of a world and a mind on the basis of a history of the variety of actions that a being in the world performs" (1991, 9). Enaction theory thus allies itself with phenomenological philosophy and implicitly also with cultural anthropology, since it allows a place for culture in the production of cognition. The crucial phrase in their formulation is "a being in the world," a phrase deliberately in resonance with phenomenological thinking. In another turn of phrase they explain that they wish to be able to reconcile the study of cognition with the fact of human experience, of subjectivity and intentionality. This leads to problems with the concept of the self as a unified entity (which they call the "I of the storm" in their chap. 4), to which I will return later.

A further aspect of cognitivism is its concentration on cognition as "problem solving." Even within this sphere it runs into difficulties, however. It proves very hard, for example, to develop robotic programs based on artificial intelligence that can simulate commonsense knowledge such as driving along a street in a car. Such a difficulty suggests that human thinking does not simply operate as a robot does. As Varela and his colleagues note, in the 1970s workers in cognitive science realized that "even the simplest cognitive action requires a seemingly infinite amount of knowledge, which we take for granted" (1991, 148). I may add here, as I write this section in a small town in Germany, Lörrach, near to the borders with both Switzerland and France, that whenever one moves into a new environment there has to be a resocialization of the body into an understanding of practices that are subtly different from one another, and the effort to do so brings into consciousness the amount of knowledge one needs simply in order to get about anywhere in a complex and structured environment. Nor can one be comfortable again until the new knowledge has been converted into a series of bodily habits. Humans seem to be able to achieve this kind of transition in a period of days, whereas digitally based machines cannot easily simulate the process, because of the "unmanageable ambiguity" of backgrounds. Cognitivism therefore pushes this problem into the periphery; we should restore it, however, to the center of the study of action and regard context-dependent know-how as the "very essence of—creative—cognition" (148).

Cognition thus becomes the "enactment," or "bringing forth," of meaning from a background of existing understandings. The process of enactment thus allows for variability and for relativity, and the concept is seen to be similar to the idea of hermeneutics, as developed by Gadamer: the bringing forth, or creation of, meaning from a variety of sources, textual or otherwise. The gestalt concept of the relationship between figure and background is also relevant here. Varela and his colleagues closely parallel this gestalt idea when they speak of inter-

pretation as "the enactment of a domain of distinctions out of a background" (1991, 156). In creating such enactments, the human brain does
not work in the same input-output way as a digital computer does.
With the computer "the meaning of a given keyboard sequence is
always assigned by the designer," but with living systems interaction
"is the result of the organization and history of the system itself" (157).
It is for this reason that the model of neural networks has replaced earlier image schemata of how the brain works, and the structure of
embodied perception becomes the starting point for analysis—e.g., of
the phenomenon of color—rather than supposed characteristics of a
pre-given world outside of perception (167). On the other hand, color
perception does not vary randomly in the cross-cultural record: there
are certain basic color terms, and, even if these are not present in a
given language, speakers of that language find it easier to learn and
remember basic rather than peripheral categories (a finding made by
Rosch in her research with the Dani people of Irian Jaya) (169). Fuzzy
set intersections provide intermediate categories of colors, and there is
cultural variability in how many of these derived categories are perceived. Therefore, color categorization depends on "a tangled hierarchy" of processes, some common to our species, some culturally specific, and it constitutes a domain that is "experiential and enacted"
(171). "Experiential" here is an interactionist concept, specifying that
cognition is neither simply the recovery of a pre-given world, as in the
realist view, nor the projection of an inner world, as in idealism. The
concept of cognition as "embodied action" is offered as a means of
bypassing—or we might say transcending—the inner-outer dichotomy. The authors recognize clearly that this idea was expressed earlier
by Merleau-Ponty (173).

    In cognitive studies the research program that emerges from this
starting point of embodied action stresses that enaction is specific but
not arbitrary. Basic levels of categorization are found that correspond
to both meaning and function as validated in cultural experience. These
basic categories, in turn, correspond to the kinesthetic image schemata
proposed by Mark Johnson—for example, the container schema, with
its basic inside-outside logic. These schemata are seen by Johnson as
arising out of basic sensorimotor activities, and their further projections
are "themselves motivated by the structures of bodily experience"
(Varela et al. 1991, 178).

    How are such insights to be applied in cultural anthropology?

Enaction, as we have seen, is virtually the same as embodiment, although given a cognitive slant, and image schemata in Johnson's work are mechanisms or instantiations of enaction/embodiment. All three concepts therefore overlap and reinforce one another. Taken together, they begin to provide a perspective on knowledge, experience, and consciousness that can deepen our view of both semantics and the character of human social action. Knowledge in this viewpoint is not statically located in some organic or superorganic sphere. It is, rather, always "enacted in particular situations" (Varela et al. 1991, 179).

This position is close to that taken in some versions of postmodernist anthropology. First, the idea that the world is not pre-given and that everything we know is therefore in some sense "constructed" fits with the antifoundationalism and "incredulity towards metanarratives" with which the postmodernist viewpoint was launched by Rorty, Lyotard, and others. The associated return to specific, local narratives (*petits récits,* in Lyotard's terms) also constitutes the revived significance of ethnography in postmodernist writings. Third, there is an apparent fit also with the stress on experimental forms of writing, which themselves become icons of enaction, particular ways of writing used to bring out particular aspects of a situation being discussed. Yet, the precise position taken by Varela and his colleagues is emphatically not one that leads to an "anything goes" approach nor to extreme subjectivism/solipsism/nihilism, as found in more extreme versions of postmodernist texts. On the contrary, by arguing that cognition is a complex of species-specific and culture-specific patterns, they return us to the project of cross-cultural comparisons on which earlier versions of anthropology were based, but this time with a more sophisticated psychological perspective. In cross-cultural cognitive studies, for example, the aim would become to see how situated enaction corresponds at another level to more general schemata. This same viewpoint can be applied also to Csordas's analysis of religious experience. Demonic possession, for example, begins with an inchoate (pre-objective) feeling of loss of control over the body and its intentional movements (its sensorimotor coherence). This is then objectified by a healer in terms of what Johnson calls the "container schema" and is diagnosed as an intrusion across a boundary, to be corrected by a suitable form of embodied action in response. What emerges, then, is both something quite particular and also something comparable to other contexts in which the container schema is similarly activated. We are not dealing here only with semantics, either, since we are looking at ritual actions undertaken as therapy to alter a person's consciousness and therefore the social relationships that flow from this consciousness. Csordas's use of the distinction between the pre-objective and the objectified seems very useful here as a means of enabling us to see how enaction is both generated and accomplished.

It is evident, also, that the level of action that is here being theorized is primarily that of the individual, albeit the culturally situated individual. Somewhat paradoxically, another aspect of the work by Varela and his colleagues is precisely that they are led to question the idea of the unitary self that lies at the back of some senses of this term *individual*. In pursuing the concept of embodiment, it now becomes important to face this problem.

Varela and his colleagues do so in their chapter called "The I of the Storm," with the subtitle "What Do We Mean by Self?" It is important to notice that they approach this question in terms of the brain and its operations rather than from the point of view of cultural categories and that they proceed also from an ethnophenomenolgy of perception and sensation. Yet they turn also to Buddhist philosophy in order to show that in some traditions of thought the self is *not* essentialized or considered transcendent; rather the tendency to cling to the idea of the self is criticized. From this tradition also they draw a critique of the concept of consciousness, noting that it alone cannot be the basis for an idea of a unitary self because of the momentary and unconnected character of the stream of consciousness or awareness (here it seems they may be neglecting the aspect of memory). Following Buddhist traditions, they conclude that "cognition and experience do not appear to have a truly existing self" and also that "the habitual belief in such an ego-self . . . is the basis of the origin and continuation of human suffering" (Varela et al. 1991, 80). This "finding" they take to be the counterpart within the mind itself of the "Cartesian anxiety" about the outside world about whether it really exists apart from our own cognition of it. The self does not exist other than as the outcome of aggregate processes within the brain and the world is shaped by, as well as shaping, our cognitive processes. From this emerges their notion of "selfless minds" (106–30), a picture closely related to Minsky's propositions in his book *Society of Mind* (1986; cited in ibid., 107). Minsky argues that action results from the combination of a multitude of actions by agents and that this also is the process that occurs between neural networks in the brain. The notion that there is a self behind all these events he regards as humanistic myth but one that we cannot apparently do without. As Varela and his colleagues note, this condemns us to a kind of perpetual schizophrenia, because of "an unbridgeable contradiction between cognitive science and human experience" (129). Minsky's conclusions are similar to those of Jackendoff in *Consciousness and the Computational Mind* (125–26). For Jackendoff the computational mind, which operates largely without the necessity for awareness, is basic, and consciousness is simply a curious (i.e., unexplained) "amalgam of the effects on the mind of both thought and the real world" (126). Consciousness for both Minsky and Jackendoff is thus an anomaly.

In effect, Varela and his colleagues appear both to agree and disagree with Minsky and Jackendoff. They agree in denying that there is any true self. They disagree in that they wish to propose the concept of embodiment as their solution to the problem of the self. "We" are embodied beings, they say. It is our embodiment that is our true character. Embodiment is thus the master concept to cut the Gordian knot regarding self/not-self, and mediated perception is the basis of all knowledge.

From an anthropological point of view, as I have briefly hinted, such a conclusion is both useful and insufficient. First, there is the matter of cultural categories. Self, as they themselves note, is handled differently in different historical and philosophical traditions. Self, in fact, *is* a cultural category. As such, it cannot be "disproved," since it exists in the cultural and social realm, regardless of whether it does or does not correspond to some features of "the brain." Second, from within phenomenological philosophy embodiment includes "memory," and it is this memory that constitutes, to a great extent, identity. The embodied person, as Merleau-Ponty notes, is a portmanteau of memories that constitute a complex configuration of identities, within which self has its place along with other aspects. And the organization of these aspects varies culturally. The anthropologist thus "bypasses" the problem of the self differently from the psychologist—not by denying it but by objectifying and relativizing it.

Naomi Quinn has made similar points in her examination of the joint work by Lakoff and Johnson on metaphor. Quinn comments on the idea that metaphor is a mapping from a source onto a target domain (1991, 57) and that such mappings are a result of the transposition of originally embodied image schemata. She accepts that mappings of this kind may partially underlie our process of understanding but points out that where they do so, they operate within the frameworks of particular *cultural* patterns or predispositions. Metaphors are chosen for their match with findings from her research with American couples regarding marriage, which suggest the abstract ideas of sharing, benefit, and compatibility underlying people's responses. These ideas are then taken by her as constitutive and as nonmetaphorical.

Perhaps Quinn and Lakoff/Johnson are talking past each other in this debate. Quinn's insistence on the constitutive role of culture is certainly correct. Lakoff and Johnson's image schemata contain large amounts of cultural "materials" and might have to be established anew in each cultural case before one could generalize or talk about universals. They might, however, reply to Quinn's objections that the abstract concepts she discusses tend to be expressed in image schematic terms—e.g., sharing as "being together," benefit as "balance," compatibility as "fit." Quinn herself, at the end of her paper, admits that "what the underlying structure of cultural models is, if not metaphoric or image schematic, I am not prepared to say" (1991, 93). Perhaps they are all culture specific. Meanwhile, Lakoff and Johnson have set us a problem to investigate further.

A different kind of issue has been raised by Roger Keesing (n.d.). Keesing notes the universalism-relativism dilemma (22) and suggests that universals may provide pathways for particulars. As I have done, he appeals to the phenomenological studies of embodiment here. But he notes the danger of the intrusion of ideology into our theory. What about power and gender? Images of embodiment are likely to be gendered (as they are notably, e.g., among the Kabyle studied by Pierre Bourdieu). Image schemata are available for use at the praxis level in motivated ways, and "when . . . speakers choose among these resources and deploy them, inequalities of power are played out" (20). Discourse may entail the hegemonic imposition of such schemata. Keesing thus draws us back to a field of interpretation more familiar to anthropologists since the impact of Marxist thought on anthropology: the role of ideology. Putting Foucault in tandem with Merleau-Ponty would give us the same result, albeit by a different, Maussian, pathway (*"les techniques du corps"*).

Quinn therefore reinserts culture into the debate, and Keesing reminds us of the hegemonic aspects of cultural discourse. Neither, however, questions the basic concept of embodiment as an important source of both meaning and action. We can see, therefore, a confluence of ideas from both cognitive science and cultural anthropology that converge on this concept and, in doing so, signalize once again the mindful body that I have taken as the starting point and now the ending of my own exploration here.

The concept of embodiment is certainly "good to think with," and I will illustrate the point further with reference to Johnny Parry's essay "The End of the Body" (1989). Parry takes up the problem of how at the sacred city of Benares in India the cremation of corpses and bodybuilding by wrestlers proceed side by side. To the Western observer this appears paradoxical, but these activities simply represent moments in the cultivation of the body and the person that proceed according to a dialectic of monist and dualistic views of the person. At an abstract level this is Parry's real interest. He notes McKim Marriott's ethnosociological picture of persons in South Asia as "divisible": a viewpoint that has found its way extensively into New Guinea ethnography subsequently (see, e.g., M. Strathern 1988). Parry's purpose is to question the sharpness of the dichotomy thus proposed between "Indian" and "Western" notions. He finds abundant evidence for ideas of a monist body-mind entity in India as well as evidence for dualistic categories. Indeed, he goes further and suggests that both patterns are also found in Western culture.

Mutability and divisibility are also seen in a caste-dominated society as sources of danger and therefore function in that context as an ideology. Exactly the same can be said for New Guinea—for example, in the well-known context of ideas about menstrual dangers. What we have to do is to understand the embodied imageries of morality that run across the supposed division of them/us. Here Parry cites the Hagen idea of the body's surface showing the inner state of the person that I have been at pains to elaborate (A. J. Strathern 1981, 1994b; M. Strathern 1979). Similar ideas exist in Benares; for example, "sin" is felt to grow out in the *hair*, which must therefore be shaved off in ritual. In reading this example, I was struck by a parallel from Pangia in the New Guinea Highlands: long hair on pigs and people coupled with a lack of fat is a sign of wrongdoing or a lack of well-being, as though the person or pig had diverted his or her life-giving energy into a removable rather than a fixed part of themselves. It is the study of detailed ethnoparameters in imagery of this sort that we need to further the investigation of embodiment in both local specifics and in cross-cultural perspective.

Embodiment and Mimesis

Another productive use of an idea that essentially appeals to embodiment is to be found in the work of Michael Taussig (appropriately enough given his long-standing interest in "performance" in social action). The idea here is that of mimesis, also used by Bourdieu and many earlier theorists of magic.

Michael Taussig in his study of "Mimesis and Alterity" (1993) pursues an intriguing set of themes through the ethnography of the Cuna and other peoples of South America. Mimesis is the imitation of the other, both as a reaction and as an attempt at appropriation, an expression of identity and difference rolled into one (or two). It has emotional, artistic, and magical roots, and Taussig reminds us of the early use of the concept in the work of Frazer on sympathetic magic. He identifies the mimetic faculty as a human characteristic that grants to "the copy the character of the original the representation the power of the represented" (Taussig 1993, xviii). Through this concept he revitalizes the old descriptive tag "fetish" and recalls Adorno's remark on Walter Benjamin, that his swatting of objects awakened "the congealed life" in them (1). He also opposes his idea of the "sensuous" to the Enlightenment idea of reason (by now a much battered notion and one that is somewhat unreasonably denied its own broad fan of meanings, but that is not at issue here).

These ideas he applies first to a problem: Why did the Cuna use wooden figurines of Europeans as curing fetishes, *nuchus?* The problem is compounded by the Cuna statement that the magical power of these fetishes resides in their inner substance, in the spirit within the wood, rather than in their outer form. Why, then, carve them at all? Why, in other words, such a form of mimetic embodiment? In his first chapter Taussig raises but does not quite solve this problem. The carvings provide the means of attracting spirits into them so that they can be controlled but, he asks again, why the drive to embodiment? Surely the basic answer must lie in Cuna ethnotheories of the body as a primal source of power.

In chapter 4 Taussig returns to this question, quoting Frazer's proposition that the magician can produce effects by imitating them, the copy influencing the original. Furthermore, this copy need not be an exact one; it may often be a stylized or partial representation. Yet what counts is its point-by-point, or modeling, analogy to the original. We can in fact compare such copies to models that do not exactly represent originals but represent, rather, their structural features, as maps, recipes, scripts do. A further feature is also often found; that the copy in some way contains a part of the substance of the original (Frazer's law of contagion). Taussig cites love magic made out of body substances here (sperm, pubic hair—the examples he gives can be paralleled exactly from contemporary practices in urban contexts in Papua New Guinea). Taussig adds here another element: it is not just ethnologic that is at work but the embodied emotional expression of the one who makes the magic. It is in the drama that power lies.

In chapter 7 another element is added to the semiotic picture. The scene shifts to Tierra del Fuego and exchanges between English sailors and indigenous islanders, scarlet cloth for local supplies of food (both sides smugly pleased in the same way and for the same reason as happened in exchanges of shells for food between Australians and New Guinea Highlands in the 1930s). The color of an object given may be magical, as it was in this instance, the red cloth perceived as similar to magical red pigments used for decorating the skin. Cloth, skin, and paint may be said to form a hermeneutic circle here, of mutually implicated "copies" and "originals," expressed in what became a mimetic trade between self and other. A further mediating element is blood, since this is red and thought to be the vehicle of *purpa*, or soul, like the substance of wood.

Chapter 8 continues the quest for meaning with a return to the Cuna concept of *purpa*, thought of as a kind of copy of an original body. This is a vital key, since it helps to explain why a carved body is needed as the means to "resituate" a powerful spirit-soul. Magical words, also, create a mimetic description of objects, actions, and movements that then exemplify or create their own magical effects. Bit by bit Taussig puts together his theory in the very way he ascribes to the Cuna healers themselves in their rites. A final piece is added in chapter 13, in which he adduces a picture of a Cuna chief and his wife, he in Western she in Cuna dress. The woman's dress in this pair represents Cuna identity, authenticity, the local power of reproduction, he suggests. Women's *mola* blouses certainly did become objectified symbols of the Cuna resistance to change, while the men's assumption of Western clothes was a mimesis of an appropriative kind. The chief and his wife thus become a composite symbol of the outer and the inner, form (clothing) and substance, which *together* produce magical power. If this is right, the meaning of the *nuchus* figures is now at last released, and a component of gender imagery is at its heart, along with the recognition of the historical experience of colonialism and the control of sexual relations—since, by dressing as they did, the Cuna women signified their nonavailability to the colonialists, whereas their men's clothes signified a mimetic appropriation as well as a new socialization of the male body to the rules of colonial hierarchy. Taussig has opened up here the history of clothing in colonial contact as well as achieving closure on the problem with which he opened his book.

But, if these findings are heuristically clear, the various meanings of the term *embodiment* and its analytical status as a concept still need to be explored further.

Embodiment: Conceptual Paradigm or Heuristic Tool?

I begin here with a rueful anecdote. In June 1994 I was giving a lecture to a research group at the Centre National de Recherches Scientifiques (CNRS) led by Daniel de Coppet. My topic was the relationship between trance and healing (see chap. 7), and I drew freely on words and phrases that have become common stock in anthropology in the last few years, including the term *embodiment*. André Iteanu, who was listening intently, interrupted me to ask what this term meant, as he found it puzzling. Surprised, I realized that I too found it puzzling, if not impossible, to give any succinct definition at all; I perceived and shared with my questioner his difficulty. Embodiment has to do with the body, but it implies that it is something else, other than or added to the physical body itself, that *is* embodied, and such a "thing" often turns out to be an abstract social value, such as honor or bravery. Embodiment thus has to do with values that in some ways are also disembodied or may be thought of separately from the body itself. *Embodiment*, in other words, is a term that belies itself by combining the abstract and the concrete together (see Ots 1994, 117).

This vignette (itself locally situated, or embodied, if you will) points to a complexity in usage that is at the heart of the problem of understanding what significance to attribute to embodiment as a concept in contemporary anthropological theorizing. The problem arises from the fact that, as the term has become more popular, its meaning has been stretched in different directions. What is inside the envelope of meaning now, then, may be quite amorphous and thus not particularly useful. The envelope has been pushed in two contradictory ways, in fact, one stressing the physical and material, the other a more mental and abstract sense of the term. A dialectic between these senses is understandable, but we have to identify where particular authors' usages stand along the continuum.

Parallel to this problem is that of the definitions of *body* itself. In some cultures such a holistic concept, implicitly in the European tradition opposed to "soul" or "spirit," may not exist. In academic writings about the body there is, in fact, a proliferation of bodies. It was Emile Durkheim who introduced into anthropology the specific notion of "homo duplex," the human being who has both a physical (for Durkheim, individual) and a spiritual (for Durkheim, social) aspect (Durkheim 1965, 306). Mary Douglas adapted this idea to her own uses by speaking of "the two bodies," physical and social, and arguing that the latter influences how we perceive the former (Douglas 1970; see chap. 2 here). Lock and Scheper-Hughes carried the process further by identifying three bodies: the individual, the social, and the body politic (1987). The picture was presented in a more complex way by John O'Neill's book, *Five Bodies,* in which he writes first of "our two bodies," by which he means "the physical" and "the communicative body" (1985, 16), and he goes on to distinguish further the world's body (the world seen on the model of the human body), social bodies, the body politic, consumer bodies, and medical bodies (chaps. 2–5). Finally, Csordas has noted (in the foreword to his 1994 edited collection) that in postmodernist times the concept of the body has become complex and multiple, essentially resisting definitions. I am not taking issue with these presentations as such but only note that the list is in principle extendable in any direction we choose (e.g., the sexual body, the aging body, the prosthetic body, the suffering body), and this without much theoretical advancement beyond seeing how many aspects of human experience can be powerfully conveyed by concentrating on the body. It is important also to recognize that the physical body is required as a silent, unmarked category in all of these usages. Medical bodies are physical bodies seen from a particular angle, and so are all the other categories. Yet the physical or biological body carries little meaning *unless* it is seen through some other aspect, and hence the term *embodiment* comes into its own. What is embodied is always some set of meanings, values, tendencies, orientations, that derive from the sociocultural realm.

But it is equally important to see that in many instances these meanings are expressed only, or at least most clearly, in an embodied form. They may, of course, be expressed also in aesthetic genres that become objectifications of experience and in turn influence it. The body may be a symbol among other symbols. Notable here also is the fact that *embodiment* is being used to refer to human beings only, and not to material artifacts. Yet we know also that such artifacts may carry powerful meanings as extensions of the human body or in being modeled on the human body (or vice versa). Hence, it is difficult simply to restrict embodiment to the living human body.

One reason why we may tend to do so is that, as I have noted, the physical human body has to enter in as a component of all the other bodies that writers may conjure up. Embodiment itself becomes a metaphor rather than a concretization when we extend it in this way. In a larger sense, though, the concentration on the human body as such may cause us to miss the ethnographic point in cultures in which the body is seen as a part of a wider cosmos, just as in an animistic context it would be a mistake to concentrate on human souls alone (even if analytically we consider the phenomena to be a result of anthropomorphic thinking).

Granted, then, that in some sense it is always the same physical human body that is said to embody different aspects of experience, it becomes possible to ask why this is such a significant matter and why its significance was not stressed so greatly in earlier phases of anthropological writings? The answer is that in recent theorizing the body has clearly been set up as a kind of baseline universal. When the sociologist Bryan Turner asks why social theorists have tended to overlook our most fundamental feature, that of embodiment, he means the fact of having a body with all the capacities and advantages as well as disadvantages (e.g., sickness, mortality) that this implies. He appeals to the physical end of the spectrum of meaning for the term and at the same time to the phenomenological interpretation of the physical as specificity, situatedness, perspective. Yet, since what is embodied is clearly not just the physical but the social and cultural as well (consider Bour-

dieu's habitus), the body as baseline also turns into the body as culturally relative.

In general, however, whether the body is seen as universal or as
relative, it is evident that its reentry into the scene of social theorizing
results from a reaction against mentalistic patterns of inquiry and
explanation that had previously dominated. But we must ask also why
such a reaction should have occurred. In general, I would relate this to
what postmodernist writers have pointed to as the declining persua-
siveness of modernist paradigms and their ideological underpinnings
both in social life and the work of social theorists. *Post-modernism* is, of
course, a confusing and imprecise term, covering a multitude of sins
(and perhaps a few virtues) (see, for good surveys, Rosenau 1992;
Smart 1992). But the relevance of invoking it here is to ask, when grand
theories, paradigms, or metanarratives fail, what can the analyst or
ethnographer fall back upon as a starting point or a focus for inquiry?
Theories are abstractions. If we have become suspicious of such
abstractions, what is next at hand? Obviously, our own immediate
being, which is most apparent and yet sometimes most hidden to us.
Hence, I would argue, the stress on embodiment, which constitutes as I
see it a muted universalism at the back of an emphasis on local knowledge and local constructions of the person. Embodiment is, therefore, a
new humanism, not exactly soteriological but one that is intended to
bring us back to ourselves. It is, put simply, a reaction against disem-
bodiment, a reinstallment of gemeinschaft against the gesellschaft quality of bureaucratic politics. Embodiment is a post-Weberian and post-
Marxian concept that nevertheless is able to draw on the themes of
asceticism and exploitation advanced by these two grand theorists,
seen, as it were, through the eyes of Michel Foucault. (My formulation
here has been helped by the survey in Synnott 1993, 228–64.)

That embodiment represents a return to the sensuous quality of
lived experience, and thus naturally bases itself largely on phenomenology, can be seen from the fact that along with new analyses that
stress a revised viewpoint on concepts of "the person," there is also a
spate of works that stress the senses and the bodily sites at which these
senses are activated. The ghost of David Hume looks out from behind
Descartes and Kant but this time combined with an interest in the sensuous bases of experience rather than simply as a touchstone of knowledge. This new empiricism embraces the emotions and their link with
the senses by way of vision, touch, smell, hearing. Anthony Synnott's

book is a good example of this genre. Starting with body and gender as concepts, he proceeds quickly to recognizable "sites": beauty and the face, hair, the senses, touch, smell, and sight, and a final chapter called "bodies and senses." Such an approach is good both for "bringing us back to ourselves" (out of the Cartesian cogito myth) and for stretching our imaginations to realize Hamlet's point to Horatio that "there are more things in Heaven and earth than are dreamed of in your philosophy." He cites, for example, David Maybury-Lewis's anecdote on the Xavante of Brazil, in which after shamanistic healing dances the people heard the souls of the dead whistling around them; and Paul Stoller's account of how he failed to experience a man's spirit double sought by a *sorko* healer among the Songhay of Niger (Synnott 1993, 153). Stoller himself has articulated a clear general position of what he calls radical empiricism based on the senses in his book *The Taste of Ethnographic Things: The Senses in Anthropology* (1989).

Many field workers in anthropology can recover memories that would contribute to this theme and belong also to the area of inquiry that has to do with altered states of consciousness. In my own case I vividly recall how I was sleeping in a camp bed in my field house in Mount Hagen (Papua New Guinea) and was woken up by a knocking at the woven-cane outer wall of the house next to my ear and the voice of a close acquaintance of mine, who I thought was hundreds of miles away in the capital city of Port Moresby. He was saying, "Andrew, I have come." Outside there was no one to be seen, but I was told that my friend had been brought up by a hospital car at night and had died (of cancer) just before dawn. What to make of such experiences? They challenge either our epistemologies or our knowledge of the power of our senses. For the peoples we study, however, they represent common sense itself. Of course, the Hageners assured me, my friend's spirit came to greet me just at the point of his death, and the spirit is not so much disembodied as a replica in a transformed way of the living person. Such examples demand that we take most seriously local theories of embodiment/disembodiment, at the very least in order to understand what the local common sense is (see Badone 1995; Salamone 1995). The study of such experiences is also helpful as a means of understanding how local ideas reproduce and transform themselves over time, whether we explain them as hypnagogic hallucinations or as "real" manifestations of some sort. Accounts of them also reveal the construction of "memories."

Whether we adopt the radical relativism that is suggested by such impressionistic anecdotes from the cross-cultural record or not, it is impossible in any case not to acknowledge the impact of books that are turning embodiment in the direction of the senses as a means of revitalizing ethnography itself (see, e.g., Ackerman 1990; Howes 1991; Classen 1993; Classen, Howes, and Synnott 1994; Seremetakis 1994). The challenging collection of essays in Seremetakis, for example, stretches experience beyond the human body to include "the dense communication between persons and things" in the context of memory and history. Seremetakis sets up the category of "sensory memory" as

> a cultural form not limited to the psychic apparatus of a monadic, pre-cultural and a historical subject but embedded and embodied in a dispersed surround of created things, surfaces, depths, and densities that are stratigraphic sites of sensory biography and history, (descr. of the book [1994, 147]).

Brief reflection can show that this, too, is a way of bringing us back to the immediacy of our own lives, since every house or home represents the creation of multiple biographical sites of this sort that gather their meanings only from being perceived and used. In other cultures such sensory biographies may be differently inscribed—for instance, in named small localities and their associations (as is done commonly in the New Guinea Highlands, e.g., in which a complex web of locality names is linked to personal experiences as well as being the foundational grid of rights to land and house sites). In fact, this way of looking at material culture may serve to remind us of the viewpoint propounded by Marcel Mauss on the relationship between persons and things: that things may themselves be seen as "agents" and thus as "being," in a way comparable to the being of people. Yet, as Gingrich (1994, 175–77) has pointed out, we cannot gain direct access to the experiential side of such notions: we must always be at least partly dependent on local words and concepts as our guides, for example, with regard to the experience of temporality through ritual. In a different vein, however, we can recognize the importance of developing ways of studying bodily movements by direct transcriptions such as Labanotation, as recently argued persuasively by Farnell (1994).

Viewpoints of this kind in anthropology have recently received support from trends within philosophy. Charles Taylor, for example, in his essay "To Follow a Rule" has argued for the importance of embodiment in the concept of acquiescence to social rules. In doing so, he essentially follows the approaches made by Pierre Bourdieu and others that became the foundation for practice theory. It is rules as performed, as enacted, that Taylor (1985) is interested in, taking performance as constitutive here.

A similar approach is taken by Rom Harré in his work *Physical Being* (1991). Harré follows his earlier work on the social construction of the emotions by examining their corporeal basis as "the experience of embodiment." Rejecting scientific classification of body parts as the measure against which to consider cultural categorizations, he notes the symbolic significance attributed to the left and right hands in many cultures and suggests that many other ways of ordering dimensions (e.g., upper/lower) may also be relevant. On the emotions he distinguishes between "haptic" feelings, based on touching, and "hedonic" feelings, ones that give pleasure or pain. Haptic feelings instantiate the reversibility of perception because of the possibility of touching oneself, as Merleau-Ponty argued (Harré 1991, 95). Hedonic feelings are constructionist: whatever is brought together as pleasurable or painful becomes so (98). Here Harré makes the familiar observation that pain is expressed differently in different cultures, from very low-key to very melodramatic. One could add here that the valorization of pain can vary greatly, and it must be seen as "human experience" that is culturally situated (for a detailed exposition, see Good et al. 1992). Finally, here Harré turns to the experience of embodiment in skilled bodily actions that are the product of training. As he points out, from the observer's viewpoint the impression is one of smoothness and economy, features that are experienced by the performer simply as "getting it right." In either case, however, the experience is holistic, what Merleau-Ponty calls *"praktognosia,"* corresponding to approaches to action known nowadays as praxiological. In a later chapter he turns to inscriptional meanings of the body, similar to those I have explored in chapter 4, calling these "corporeal semantics." Interestingly, he takes one of his examples from the Hua people of New Guinea, with their concept of *nu*, or vital substance, attached differently to the genders but a common focus of their interest. When philosophy comes to ethnography, we know that the wheel has indeed turned away from the *cogito* into the embodied *sum*.

Embodiment as an Analytical Concept

But, if all this is so, there is also a need to delineate the precise analytical position that the concept of embodiment has in this new form of ethnography (a form that can be seen as post-postmodern, or simply as "reconstructive"). I have already indicated that the term has two poles of meaning, corresponding broadly to the ideas of the physical and the social body developed by Mary Douglas out of Durkheim's original attempt to explain the body-soul dichotomy. A somewhat more complicated picture of the discursive field now needs to be constructed, in which the strategic place of the term *embodiment* can be visualized. I see it as a mediating term between two different anthropologies, which we may conceptualize as being based on nouns in one case and verbs in the other, as follows:

Nouns	→→→→	*Verbs*
Society	E	Action
	M	
Person	B	Practice
	O	
Individual/Dividual	D	Experience
	I	
Self	M	Enactment
	E	
Consciousness	N	Representation
	T	
CoPresence		Communication

Embodiment in this sense is a transformer, or transducer, enabling us to move back and forth between noun-based and verb-based concepts while recognizing that the historical movement is from nouns to verbs (represented by the arrow in my scheme). The stress is thus on action and performance, on doing rather than being, or on the being that resides in doing, that issues from and is expressed only in doing. Performativity is made central to social life generally, not just as a characteristic of certain societies or cultures as in Marshall Sahlins's characterization of Hawaii (1985).

The idea of embodiment can also be used to concretize discussions of the self. There are problems, however, with the term *self* because of its inextricable involvement with psychological theorizing. Such problems emerge, for example, in Nancy Rosenberger's edited collection *Japanese Sense of Self* (1992), in which the concepts discussed depart so markedly from ideas of an internal, unique individual that they would be better signalized by another roster of terms. One of the more notable attempts to re-empower the concept of selfhood in spite of this sort of "semantic contamination" has been made by Thomas Csordas. Csordas has brought his thinking to culmination in his book *The Sacred Self* (1994). Here he builds on his earlier essay (1990) on embodiment as a paradigm by explicating the notion of self in phenomenological terms as a kind of orientation toward the world in a field marked by the co-presence of others. This conceptualization marks precisely the movement from being to doing (or, equally, becoming) that I have incorporated into my diagram. Csordas blends the idea of copresence with a theory of ritual akin to that of Catherine Bell (1992) in order to argue that the orientational self is constructed by means of a picture of the other as not-self but that communication with this other is what constitutes the sacred self. Whether one fully accepts this analysis or not, the notion of embodiment enables Csordas powerfully to focus on the actual rituals and interactions performed by the Catholic Charismatics whom he studied and to bring out the bodily, kinesthetic components in their constructions of religious meanings.

It is abundantly evident, then, that embodiment is *at least* a creative heuristic tool for this and many other inquiries. It would become paradigmatic if a set of propositions about social life were to emerge from its use in research that would command wide agreement among practitioners. Here I use *paradigmatic* not to refer to a set of explanatory theories but in terms of "guiding orientations" that are implicitly accepted. In this sense it may be only a matter of time before *embodiment* achieves centrality in social inquiries. The question then will be "How long will it stay in that position?" and the answer will depend simply on what is invested (or embodied) in the concept itself. My suggestion has been, in effect, that the term represents a kind of hybrid, a heuristic protoparadigm that enables us to make a bridge from one broad set of perspectives in social thought to another. As a hybrid looking both ways, it is perhaps preeminently suited to a historical period in which established dichotomies no longer work and the modernist/postmodernist debate, particularly, has run its course. As Bruno Latour (1994) might have put it, we may never have been modern—but we have always been, and always will be, embodied, regardless of our latest attempts to achieve a disembodied existence by means of the Internet and cyberspace—a theme that is well portrayed in the medium of science fiction writing itself by the novels of William Gibson (see, e.g., 1987), in which great poignancy resides in the juxtaposition of the emotional and physical fragility of humans and the frighteningly powerful machines that they create and into whose "world" they enter. The theme of embodiment is an attempt to return to conditions of our being that tend to be obliterated by the objectifications of late-capitalist technology. Its useful employment as an analytical term in anthropological theorizing is thus shadowed by its dialectical relationship with the wider social currents into which such theorizing is set.

References

Ackerman, Diane. 1990. *A Natural History of the Senses*. New York: Random House.

Allen, N. J. 1985. The category of the person: a reading of Mauss's last essay. In *The Category of the Person*, ed. M. Carrithers et al, 26–45. Cambridge: Cambridge University Press.

Atkinson, Jane Monnig. 1989. *The Art and Politics of Wana Shamanship*. Berkeley: University of California Press.

———. 1992. Shamanisms today. *Annual Reviews in Anthropology* 21:307–30.

Austin, J. L. 1962. *How to Do Things with Words*. Oxford: Oxford University Press.

Badone, Ellen. 1995. Suspending disbelief: an encounter with the occult in Brittany. *Anthropology and Humanism* 20(1): 9–14.

Barrett, Robert J., and Rodney H. Lucas. 1993. The skulls are cold, the house is hot: interpreting depths of meaning in Iban therapy. *Man*, n.s., 28(3): 573–96.

Barth, Fredrik. 1975. *Ritual and Knowledge among the Baktaman of New Guinea*. Oslo: Universitetsforlaget.

Battaglia, Debbora, ed. 1995. *Rhetorics of Self-Making*. Berkeley: University of California Press.

Baudinet, Marie-José. 1989. The face of Christ, the form of church. In *Fragments for a History of the Human Body*, ed. M. Feher, R. Naddaff, and N. Tazi, 148–56. New York: ZONE.

Baudrillard, Jean. 1993. *Symbolic Exchange and Death*. Trans. I. H. Grant. London: Sage Publications.

Beauvoir, Simone De. 1949. *Le Deuxième sexe 1: les faits et les mythes*. Paris: Édition Gallimard.

Bell, Catherine. 1992. *Ritual Theory, Ritual Process*. Berkeley: University of California Press.

Bettelheim, Bruno. [1954] 1962. *Symbolic Wounds, Puberty Rites and the Envious Male*. New York: Collier Press.

Biersack, Aletta. 1982. Ginger gardens for the ginger woman: rites and passages in a Melanesian society. *Man*, n.s., 17: 239–58.

———. 1983. Bound blood: Paiela "conception theory" interpreted. *Mankind* 14: 85–100.

Blackburn, Julia. 1979. *The White Men: The First Response of Aboriginal People to the White Man.* London: Orbis Publishing.

Bloch, Maurice. 1986. *From Blessing to Violence: History and Ideology in the Circumcision Ritual of the Merina of Madagascar.* Cambridge: Cambridge University Press.

Boddy, Janice. 1989. *Wombs and Alien Spirits.* Toronto: University of Toronto Press.

Bonnemère, Pascale. 1992. Le casoar, le pandanus rouge, et l'anguille. Ph.D. diss., École des Hautes Études en Sciences Sociales (EHESS), Paris.

Bourdieu, Pierre. 1977. *Outline of the Theory of Practice.* Trans. Richard Nice. Cambridge: Cambridge University Press.

————. 1984. *Distinction: A Social Critique of the Judgement of Taste.* Trans. Richard Nice. Cambridge, Mass.: Harvard University Press.

Bourguignon, Erika, ed. 1973. *Religion, Altered States of Consciousness, and Social Change.* Columbus: Ohio State University Press.

Brown, Paula, and G. Buchbinder, eds. 1976. *Man and Woman in the New Guinea Highlands.* Spec. Pub. no. 8. American Anthropological Association.

Brown, Peter. 1988. *The Body and Society. Men, Women, and Sexual Renunciation in Early Christianity.* New York: Columbia University Press.

Buckley, Thomas, and Alma Gottlieb, eds. 1988. Introduction. *Blood Magic: The Anthropology of Menstruation,* 3–50. Berkeley: University of California Press.

Bulmer, Ralph N. H. 1965. The Kyaka of the Western Highlands. In *Gods, Ghosts and Men in Melanesia,* ed. P. Lawrence and M. J. Meggitt, 132–61. Melbourne: Oxford University Press.

Burke, Kenneth. 1961. *The Rhetoric of Religion.* Berkeley: University of California Press.

————. 1966. *Language as Symbolic Action.* Berkeley: University of California Press.

————. 1973. *The Philosophy of Literary Form.* Berkeley: University of California Press.

Burridge, Kenelm. 1979. *Someone, No-One: An Essay on Individuality.* Princeton, N.J.: Princeton University Press.

Butler, Judith. 1993. *Bodies that Matter: On the Discursive Limits of "Sex."* Routledge: London and New York.

Bynum, Caroline Walker. 1989. The female body and religious practice in the later Middle Ages. In *Fragments for a History of the Human Body,* ed. M. Feher, R. Naddaff, and N. Tazi, pt. 1: 160–219. New York: ZONE Press.

————. 1994. *The Resurrection of the Body in Western Christianity, 200–1336.* New York: Columbia University Press.

Cannon, Walter B. [1915] 1963. *Bodily Changes in Pain, Hunger, Fear and Rage.* New York: Harper and Row Publishers.

Carrier, James. 1992. *History and Tradition in Melanesian Anthropology.* Berkeley: University of California Press.

Carrithers, M., et al., eds. 1985. *The Category of the Person: Anthropology, Philosophy, History.* Cambridge and New York: Cambridge University Press.

Classen, Constance. 1993. *Worlds of Sense*. London: Routledge.

Classen, Constance, David Howes, and Anthony Synnott. 1994. *Aroma: The Cultural History of Smell*. London and New York: Routledge.

Cohen, Anthony P. 1994. *Self Consciousness: An Alternative Anthropology of Identity*. London: Routledge.

Collier, J. F., and M. Z. Rosaldo. 1981. Politics and gender in simple societies. In *Sexual Meanings: The Cultural Construction of Gender and Sexuality*, ed. S. B. Ortner and H. Whitehead. Cambridge: Cambridge University Press.

Connerton, Paul. 1989. *How Societies Remember*. Cambridge: Cambridge University Press.

Connor, Linda H. 1990. Seances and spirits of the dead: context and idiom in symbolic healing. *Oceania* 60(1): 345–59.

Conrad, Peter, and Joseph Schneider. 1992. *Deviance and Medicalization: From Badness to Sickness*, new ed., Philadelphia: Temple University Press.

Cottingham, John, ed. 1992. *The Cambridge Companion to Descartes*. Cambridge: Cambridge University Press.

Craib, Ian. 1990. *Psychoanalysis and Social Theory*. Amherst: University of Massachusetts Press.

Crapanzano, Vincent. 1992. *Hermes' Dilemma and Hamlet's Desire: on the Epistemology of Interpretation*. Cambridge, Mass.: Harvard University Press.

Csordas, Thomas. 1990. Embodiment as a paradigm for anthropology. *Ethos* 18: 5–47.

———. 1994a. *The Sacred Self: A Cultural Phenomenology of Charismatic Healing*. Berkeley: University of California Press.

———, ed. 1994b. *Embodiment and Experience: The Existential Ground of Culture and Self*. Cambridge: Cambridge University Press.

Damasio, Antonio R. 1994. *Descartes' Error*. New York: G. P. Putnam's Sons.

Delaney, Carole. 1986. The meaning of paternity and the virgin birth debate. *Man*, n.s. 21(3): 494–513.

———. 1987. Seeds of honor, fields of shame. In *Honor, Shame and the Unity of the Mediterranean*, ed. D. Gilmore, 35–48. Washington, D.C.: American Anthropological Association Publishing.

Desjarlais, Robert R. 1989. Healing through images: the magical flight and healing geography of Nepali shamans. *Ethos* 17(3): 289–307.

———. 1992. *Body and Emotion: The Aesthetics of Illness and Healing in the Nepal Himalayas*. Philadelphia: University of Pennsylvania Press.

Douglas, M. 1970. *Natural Symbols: Explorations in Cosmology*. New York: Pantheon Books (Random House).

———. [1966] 1984. *Purity and Danger: An Analysis of the Concepts of Pollution and Taboo*. London: ARK Paperbacks (Routledge and Kegan Paul).

Dow, James. 1986. Universal aspects of symbolic healing: a theoretical synthesis. *American Anthropologist*, 88: 56–69.

Durkheim, Emile, [1915] 1965. *The Elementary Forms of the Religious Life*. New York: Free Press.

Easterling, P. E., and J. V. Muir, eds. 1985. *Greek Religion and Society*. Cambridge: Cambridge University Press.

Elias, Norbert. 1982. *The Civilizing Process.* Trans. E. Jephcott. 2 vols. Oxford: Blackwell.

Erickson, Milton. 1980. *The collected papers of Milton H. Erickson on Hypnosis.* Ed. Ernest Rossi. 3 vols. New York: Irvington Press.

Farnell, Brenda M. 1994. Ethno-graphics and the moving body. *Man,* n.s., 29(4): 929–974.

Favazza, Armando R., M.D., and Barbara Favazza, M.D. 1992. *Bodies under siege: Self-Mutilation in Culture and Psychiatry.* Baltimore and London: Johns Hopkins University Press.

Featherstone, Mike, Mike Hepworth and Bryan S. Turner, eds. 1991. *The Body: Social Process and Cultural Theory.* London: Sage Publications.

Felman, Shoshana. 1987. *Jacques Lacan and the Adventure of Insight.* Psychoanalysis in Contemporary Culture Series. Cambridge, Mass.: Harvard University Press.

Fernandez, James. ed. 1991. *Beyond Metaphor: The Theory of Tropes in Anthropology.* Stanford: Stanford University Press.

Finkler, Kaja. 1985. *Spiritualist Healers in Mexico: Successes and Failures of Alternative Therapeutics.* South Hadley, Mass: Bergin and Garvey Publishers.

———. 1994. *Women in Pain: Gender and Morbidity in Mexico.* Philadelphia: University of Pennsylvania Press.

Foster, George, and Barbara Anderson. 1978. *Medical Anthropology.* New York: Alfred A. Knopf.

Foucault, Michael. 1979. *Discipline and Punish: The Birth of the Prison.* Trans. A. Sheridan. Harmondsworth: Penguin Books.

———. [1978] 1990. *History of Sexuality,* vols. 1 and 2. Trans. Robert Hurley. New York: Vintage Books (Random House).

Fournier, Marcel. 1994. *Marcel Mauss.* Paris: Fayard.

Frankel, Stephen. 1986. *The Huli Response to Illness.* Cambridge: Cambridge University Press.

Frankel, Stephen, and Gilbert Lewis, eds. 1989. *A Continuing Trial of Treatment: Medical Pluralism in Papua New Guinea.* Dordrecht: Kluwer Academic Publishers.

Frecska, E., and Z. Kulcsar. 1989. Social bonding in the modulation of the physiology of ritual trance. *Ethos* 17(1): 70–87.

Gallagher, C., and Thomas Laqueur, eds. 1987. *The Making of the Modern Body.* Berkeley: University of California Press.

Gallop, Jane. 1993. *Reading Lacan.* Ithaca, N.Y.: Cornell University Press.

Gell, Alfred. 1993. *Wrapping in Images: Tattooing in Polynesia.* Oxford: Oxford University Press.

Gewertz, Deborah. 1984. The Tchambuli view of persons: a critique of individualism in the works of Mead and Chodorow. *American Anthropologist* 86:615–29.

———. 1988. *Myths of Matriarchy Reconsidered,* Oceania Monograph no. 33. Australia: University of Sydney Press.

Gibson, William. 1987. *Count Zero.* New York: Ace Books.

Gillison, Gillian. 1993. *Between Culture and Fantasy: A New Guinea Highlands Mythology*. Chicago: University of Chicago Press.

Gingrich, André. 1994. Time, ritual and social experience. In *Social Experience and Anthropological Knowledge*, ed. Kirsten Hastrup and Peter Hervik, 166–79. London: Routledge.

Glick, Leonard B. 1963. Foundations of a primitive medical system: the Gimi of the New Guinea Highlands. Ph.D. diss., University of Pennsylvania.

———. 1967. Medicine as an ethnographic category: the Gimi of the New Guinea Highlands. *Ethnology* 6: 31–56.

Godelier, Maurice, and Marilyn Strathern, eds. 1991. *Big-Men and Great-Men: Personifications of Power in Melanesia*. Cambridge: Cambridge University Press.

Good, Mary Del Vecchio, et al., eds. 1992. *Pain as Human Experience: An Anthropological Perspective*. Berkeley: University of California Press.

Grierson, Elizabeth W. 1938. *The Scottish Fairy Book*. London: A. and C. Black.

Halbwachs, M. [1952] 1992. *On Collective Memory*. Trans. L. A. Coser. Chicago: University of Chicago Press.

Hanson, F. Allan. 1979. Does God have a body? Truth, reality and cultural relativism. *Man*, n.s., 14(3): 515–29.

Harré, Rom. 1991. *Physical Being: A Theory for a Corporeal Psychology*. Oxford: Blackwell.

Harrison, J. E. [1903] 1955. *Prolegomena to the Study of Greek Religion*. New York: Meridian Books.

———. [1921 and 1912] 1962. *Epilegomena to the Study of Greek Religion and Themis: A Study of the Social Origins of Greek Religion*. New York: University Books.

Helman, Cecil G. 1988. Psyche, soma, and society: the social construction of psychosomatic disorders. In *Biomedicine Examined*, ed. M. Lock and D. Gordon, 95–124. Dordrecht: Kluwer Academic Publishers.

Herdt, Gilbert, ed. 1982. *Rituals of Manhood: Male Initiation in Papua New Guinea*. Berkeley: University of California Press.

Héritier-Augé, Françoise. 1979. Symbolique de l'inceste et de sa prohibition. In *La Fonction symbolique: essais d'anthropologie*, ed. M. Izard and P. Smith. Paris: Gallimard.

———. 1994. *Les deux soeurs et leur mère*. Paris: Odile Jacob.

Hogan, Patrick Colm, and Lalita Pandit, eds. 1990. *Criticism and Lacan: Essays and Dialogue on Language, Structure, and the Unconscious*. Athens and London: University of Georgia Press.

Hogbin, H. Ian. 1970. *The Island of Menstruating Men: Religion in Wogeo, New Guinea*. London and Toronto: Chandler Publishing.

Hoskins, Janet. 1993. Violence, sacrifice, and divination: giving and taking life in eastern Indonesia. *American Ethnologist* 20(1): 159–178.

Howes, David, ed. 1991. *The Varieties of Sensory Experience: A Sourcebook in the Anthropology of the Senses*. Toronto: University of Toronto Press.

Johnson, Mark. 1987. *The Body in the Mind: The Bodily Basis of Meaning, Imagination, and Reason*. Chicago: University of Chicago Press.

Johnstone, Albert A. 1992. The bodily nature of the self or what Descartes should have conceded Princess Elizabeth of Bohemia. In *Giving the Body Its Due,* ed. Maxine Sheets-Johnstone, 16–47. Albany: State University of New York Press.

Jordanova, Ludmilla. 1980. Natural facts: a historical perspective on science and sexuality. In *Nature, Culture, and Gender,* ed. C. McCormack and M. Strathern, 42–69. Cambridge: Cambridge University Press.

———. 1989. *Sexual Visions.* Madison: University of Wisconsin Press.

Jorgensen, Dan. 1981. Taro and arrows: order, entropy and religion among the Telefolmin. Ph.D. diss., University of British Columbia.

———. 1983. Mirroring nature? Men's and women's models of conception in Telefolmin. Special issue ed., D. Jorgensen, *Mankind* 14(1): 57–65.

Kant, Immanuel. 1982. *Critique of Pure Reason,* trans. Wolfgang Schwarz. Aalen: Scientia Press.

Kapferer, Bruce. 1986. Performance and the structure of meaning and experience. In *The Anthropology of Experience,* ed. Victor W. Turner and Edward M. Bruner, 188–206. Chicago: University of Illinois Press.

———. 1992. Review of P. Stoller, *Fusion of the Worlds. American Ethnologist* 19(4): 845–846.

Keck, Verena. 1992. Falsch Gehandelt, Schwer Erkrankt. Kranksein bei den Yupno in Papua New Guinea, aus ethnologischer und biomedizinisches sicht. *Ethnologisches Seminar der Universität und Museum für Völkerkunde,* no. 35, Basel.

———. N.d. Two ways of explaining reality: the sickness of a little boy in Papua New Guinea from an anthropological and a biomedical point of view. Trans. Ingrid Bell-Kranhals. Ms.

Keesing, Roger M. 1992. *Custom and Confrontation: The Kwaio Struggle for Cultural Autonomy.* Chicago: University of Chicago Press.

———. N.d. The experienced body as contested site. Ms.

Kelly, Raymond. 1977. *Etoro Social Structure: A Study in Structural Contradiction.* Ann Arbor: University of Michigan Press.

———. 1993. *Constructing Inequality: The Fabrication of a Hierarchy of Virtue among the Etoro.* Ann Arbor: University of Michigan Press.

Kirmayer, Lawrence J. 1988. Mind and body as metaphors: hidden values in biomedicine. In *Biomedicine Examined,* ed. M. Lock and D. Gordon, 57–94. Dordrecht: Kluwer Academic Publishers.

Knauft, Bruce M. 1989. Bodily images in Melanesia: cultural substances and natural metaphors. In *Fragments for a History of the Human Body,* ed. M. Feher, R. Naddaff and N. Tazi, 3: 199–279. New York: ZONE Press.

Knight, Chris. 1991. *Blood Relations: Menstruation and the Origins of Culture.* New Haven and London: Yale University Press.

Kosslyn, Stephen M., and Olivier Koenig. 1992. *Wet Mind: The New Cognitive Neuroscience.* New York: Free Press.

Kramer, Fritz W. 1993. *The Red Fez: Art and Spirit Possession in Africa.* Trans. Malcolm Green. London: Verso.

Küchler, Susanne. 1992. Making skins: *Malangan* and the idiom of kinship in

Northern New Ireland. In *Anthropology, Art and Aesthetics,* ed. Jeremy Coote and Anthony Shelton, 94–111. Oxford: Clarendon Press.

Laderman, Carol. 1991. *Taming the Winds of Desire: Psychology, Medicine, and Aesthetics in Malay Shamanistic Performances.* Berkeley: University of California Press.

LaFontaine, Jean S. 1985. Person or individual: some anthropological reflections. In *The Category of the Person: Anthropology, Philosophy, History,* ed. Michael Carrithers, Steven Collins, Steven Lukes, 123–140. Cambridge: Cambridge University Press.

Lambek, Michael, 1981. *Human Spirits.* Cambridge: Cambridge University Press.

———. 1993. *Knowledge and Practice in Mayotte: Local Discourses of Islam, Sorcery, and Spirit Possession.* Toronto: University of Toronto Press.

Lancy, David. 1983. *Cross-Cultural Studies in Cognition and Mathematics.* New York: Academic Press.

Langer, Monika M. 1989. *Merleau-Ponty's Phenomenology of Perception: A Guide and Commentary.* Tallahassee: Florida State University Press.

Langness, Lew L. 1987. A day for stealing: deviance in a New Guinea society. In *Anthropology in the High Valleys,* ed. L. L. Langness and T. E. Hays, 1–26. Novato: Chandler and Sharp Publishers.

Laqueur, Thomas. 1990. *Making Sex: Body and Gender from the Greeks to Freud.* Cambridge, Mass.: Harvard University Press.

Latour, Bruno. 1994. *We Have Never Been Modern.* 2d ed. Cambridge, Mass.: Harvard University Press.

Lattas, Andrew. 1992a. Hysteria, anthropological disclosure and the concept of the unconscious: cargo cults and the scientisation of race and colonial power. *Oceania* 63(1): 1–14.

———. 1992b. Skin, personhood and redemption: the double self in West New Britain cargo cults. *Oceania* 63(1): 27–54.

LeRoy, John. 1985. *Fabricated Worlds: An Interpretation of Kewa Tales.* Vancouver: University of British Columbia Press.

Lévi-Strauss, Claude. 1969. *The Elementary Structures of Kinship.* London: Eyre and Spottiswoode.

Lewis, Gilbert. 1975. *Knowledge of Illness in a Sepik Society: A Study of the Gnau, New Guinea.* London School of Economics. Monographs on Social Anthropology, no. 52. London: Athlone Press.

———. 1980. *Day of Shining Red: An Essay on Understanding Ritual.* Cambridge: Cambridge University Press.

Lewis, Herbert S. N.d. Spirit possession today. Ms.

Liep, John. 1994. Recontextualization of a consumer good: the ritual use of Johnson's baby powder in Melanesia. In *European Imagery and Colonial History in the Pacific,* ed. Toon van Meijl and Paul van der Grijp, 64–75. Saarbrücken: Verlag für Entwicklungspolitik Breitenbach.

Lindstrom, Lamont. 1993. *Cargo Cult: Strange Stories of Desire from Melanesia and Beyond.* Honolulu: University of Hawaii Press.

LiPuma, Edward. 1988. *The Gift of Kinship: Structure and Practice in Maring Social Organization.* Cambridge: Cambridge University Press.

Lloyd, Genevieve. 1984. *The Man of Reason. "Male" and "Female" in Western Philosophy.* Minneapolis: University of Minnesota Press.

Lock, Margaret. 1993. Cultivating the body: anthropology and epistemologies of bodily practice and knowledge. *Annual Reviews in Anthropology* 22: 133–155.

Lock, Margaret, and Deborah Gordon, eds. 1988. *Biomedicine Examined.* Dordrecht: Kluwer Academic Publishing.

Lock, Margaret, and Nancy Scheper-Hughes. 1987. The mindful body. *Medical Anthropology Quarterly* 1(1): 6–41.

Lutz, Catherine. 1985. Ethnopsychology compared to what? explaining behavior and consciousness among the Ifaluk. In *Person, Self and Experience: Exploring Pacific Ethnopsychologies,* ed. Geoffrey M. White and John Fitzpatrick, 35–79. Berkeley: University of California Press.

———. 1988. *Unnatural Emotions: Everyday Sentiments on a Micronesian Atoll and Their Challenge to Western Theory.* Chicago: University of Chicago Press.

Lyotard, J.-F. 1984. *The Post-Modern Condition: A Report on Knowledge.* Minneapolis: University of Minnesota Press.

MacCormack, Carol P., and Marilyn Strathern. 1980. *Nature, Culture and Gender.* Cambridge: Cambridge University Press.

MacDonald, Mary N. 1991. *Mararoko: A Study in Melanesian Religion.* New York: Peter Lang Publishers.

Mackenzie, Maureen A. 1991. *Androgynous Objects: String Bags and Gender in Central New Guinea.* Philadelphia: Harwood Academic Publishers.

Malinowski, Bronislaw. 1922. *Argonauts of the Western Pacific.* New York: E. P. Dutton.

———. 1935. *Coral Gardens and Their Magic.* New York: American Book Company.

Martin, Emily. 1992. *The Woman in the Body: A Cultural Analysis of Reproduction,* 2d ed. Boston: Beacon Press.

———. 1994. *Flexible Bodies.* Boston: Beacon Press.

Mauss, M. 1979. *Sociology and Psychology: Essays.* Trans. B. Brewster. London: Routledge and Kegan Paul.

Mawe, Theodore. 1989. Religious cults and ritual practice among the Mendi. In *The Meaning of Things: Material Culture and Symbolic Expression,* ed. Ian Hodder, 41–49. London: Unwin Hyman.

Meggitt, Mervyn J. 1964. Male-female relations in the Highlands of Australian New Guinea. Special issue, ed. James B. Watson. *American Anthropologist* 66, (4), pt. 2: 204–24.

Meigs, Anna S. 1984. *Food, Sex and Pollution: A New Guinea Religion.* New Brunswick: Rutgers University Press.

Muller, John P., and William J. Richardson. 1982. *Lacan and Language: A Reader's Guide to Écrits.* New York: International Universities Press.

Nancy, Jean-Lue, and Phillipe Lacone-Labarthe. 1992. *The Title of the Letter: A*

Reading of Lacan. Trans. Inacore Rafford and David Pettigrew. Albany: State University of New York Press.

Narakobi, Bernard. 1982. Death of a muruk. *Bikmaus* 3(1): 72–80 (Institute of Papua New Guinea Studies, Port Moresby).

O'Hanlon, M. 1989. *Reading the Skin: Adornment, Display and Society among the Wahgi.* London: British Museum Publications.

O'Neill, John. 1985. *Five Bodies: The Human Shape of Modern Society.* Ithaca: Cornell University Press.

Onians, Richard Broxton. 1954. *The Origins of European Thought about the Body, the Mind, the Soul, the World, Time and Fate.* Cambridge: Cambridge University Press.

Ots, Thomas. 1994. The silenced body—the expressive *Leib:* on the dialectic of mind and life in Chinese cathartic healing. In *Embodiment and Experience,* ed. T. Csordas, 116–138. Cambridge: Cambridge University Press.

Padel, Ruth. 1992. *In and Out of the Mind.* Princeton, N.J.: Princeton University Press.

Panoff, Michel. 1968. The notion of double self among the Maenge. *Journal of the Polynesian Society* 77(3): 275–295.

Parker, Robert. 1983. *Miasma: Pollution and Purification in Early Greek Religion.* Oxford: Clarendon Press.

Parkin, David. 1985. *Reason, Emotion and the Embodiment of Power.* In *Reason and Morality,* ed. J. Overing. ASA monograph series 24. London: Tavistock.

Parry, J. 1989. The end of the body. In *Fragments for a History of the Human Body,* ed. M. Feher et al. pt. 2: 490–517. New York: ZONE Press.

Patterson, Mary 1974. Sorcery and witchcraft in Melanesia. *Oceania* 45: 132–60, 212–34.

Penrose, Roger. 1994. *Shadows of the Mind: A Search for the Missing Science of Consciousness.* Oxford and New York: Oxford University Press.

Poole, Fitz John Porter. 1982. The ritual forging of identity: aspects of person and self in Bimin-Kuskusmin male initiation. In *Rituals of Manhood: Male Initiation in Papua New Guinea,* ed. Gilbert Herdt. Berkeley: University of California Press.

———. 1985. Coming into social being: cultural images of infants in Bimin-Kuskusmin folk psychology. In *Person, Self and Experience: Exploring Pacific Ethnopsychologies,* ed. Geoffrey M. White and John Kirkpatrick. 183–244. Berkeley: University of California Press.

Poovey, Mary. 1987. "Scenes of an indelicate character": the medical "treatment" of Victorian women. In *The Making of the Modern Body,* ed. C. Gallagher and T. Laqueur, 137–168. Berkeley: University of California Press.

Quinn, Naomi. 1991. The cultural basis of metaphor. In *Beyond Metaphor,* ed. James Fernandez, 56–93. Stanford: Stanford University Press.

Ragland-Sullivan, Ellie. 1986. *Jacques Lacan and the Philosophy of Psychoanalysis.* Urbana and Chicago: University of Illinois Press.

Rappaport, R. A. 1979. *Ecology, Meaning and Religion.* Richmond, Calif.: North Atlantic Books.

Read, Kenneth. 1955. Morality and the concept of the person among the Gahuku-Gama. *Oceania* 25(4): 233–282.

Reay, M. O. 1959. *The Kuma: Freedom and Conformity in the New Guinea Highlands.* Melbourne: Melbourne University Press.

Rohde, Erwin. 1925. *Psyche: The Cult of Souls and Belief in Immortality among the Greeks.* London: Kegan Paul, Trench and Trubner.

Rosaldo, Michelle Z. 1980. *Knowledge and Passion: Ilongst Notions of Self and Social Life.* Cambridge: Cambridge University Press.

———. 1984. Toward an anthropology of self and feeling. In *Culture Theory,* ed. R. Shweder and R. LeVine, 137–154. Cambridge: Cambridge University Press.

Roseman, Marina. 1991. *Healing Sounds from the Malaysian Rainforest: Temiar Music and Medicine.* Berkeley: University of California Press.

Rosenau, Pauline M. 1992. *Post-modernism and the Social Sciences: Insights, Inroads, and Intrusions.* Princeton, N.J.: Princeton University Press.

Rosenberger, Nancy, ed. 1992. *Japanese Sense of Self.* Cambridge: Cambridge University Press.

Rossi, Ernest L. 1986. *The Psychobiology of Mind-Body Healing: New Concepts in Therapeutic Hypnosis.* New York: W. W. Norton.

Rossi, Ernest, and David B. Cheek. 1988. *Mind-Body Healing: Methods of Ideodynamic Healing in Hypnosis.* New York: W. W. Norton.

Rouget, Gilbert. 1985. *Music and Trance.* Chicago: University of Chicago Press.

Roustang, Francois. 1990. *The Lacanian Delusion.* Trans. Greg Sims. New York and Oxford: Oxford University Press.

Sahlins, Marshall. 1985. *Islands of History.* Chicago: University of Chicago Press.

Salamone, Frank A. 1995. The Bori and I: reflections of a mature anthropologist. *Anthropology and Humanism* 20(1): 15–19.

Salisbury, Richard F. 1965. The Siane of the Eastern Highlands. In *Gods, Ghosts and Men in Melanesia,* ed. P. Lawrence and M. J. Meggitt, 50–77. Melbourne: Oxford University Press.

Sanday, P. R. 1981. *Female Power and Male Dominance: On the Origins of Sexual Inequality.* Cambridge: Cambridge University Press.

Sarup, Madan. 1992. *Jacques Lacan.* New York: Harvester-Wheatsheaf Press.

Schiebinger, Londa. 1987. Skeletons in the closet: the first illustrations of the female skeleton in eighteenth century anatomy. In *The Making of the Modern Body,* ed. C. Gallagher and T. Laqueur, 42–82. Berkeley: University of California Press.

———. 1989. *The Mind Has No Sex? Women in the Origins of Modern Science.* Cambridge, Mass.: Harvard University Press.

———. 1993. *Nature's Body: Gender in the Making of Modern Science.* Boston: Beacon Press.

Schieffelin, Edward. 1976. *The Sorrow of the Lonely and the Burning of the Dancers.* New York: St. Martin's Press.

Seremetakis, C. Nadia, ed. 1994. *The Senses Still: Perception and Memory as Material Culture in Modernity.* New York: Westview Press.

Shaara, Lila, and Andrew Strathern 1992. A preliminary analysis of the rela-

tionship between altered states of consciousness, healing and social structure. *American Anthropologist* 94(1): 145–160.

Sheets-Johnstone, Maxine. 1994. *The Roots of Power: Animate Form and Gendered
Bodies.* Chicago: Open Court.

Shilling, Chris. 1993. *The Body and Social Theory.* London: Sage.

Shorter, Edward. 1994. *From the Mind into the Body: The Cultural Origins of Psychosomatic Symptoms.* New York: Free Press.

Silk, M. S. 1974. *Interaction in Poetic Imagery: With Special Reference to Early Greek
Poetry.* Cambridge: Cambridge University Press.

Sissa, Giulia. 1990. *Greek Virginity.* Cambridge, Mass.: Harvard University
Press.

Smart, Barry. 1993. *Postmodernity.* London: Routledge.

Stoller, Paul. 1989a. *Fusion of the Worlds: An Ethnography of Possession among the
Songhay of Niger.* Chicago: University of Chicago Press.

———. 1989b. *The Taste of Ethnographic Things: The Senses in Anthropology.*
Philadelphia: University of Pennsylvania Press.

Strathern, Andrew J. 1968. Sickness and frustration: variations in two Highlands societies. *Mankind* 6: 545–550.

———. 1971. Wiru and Daribi matrilateral payments. *Journal of the Polynesian
Society* 80: 449–462.

———. 1972. *One Father, One Blood: Descent and Group Structure among the
Melpa.* Canberra: Australian National University Press.

———. 1975. Why is shame on the skin? *Ethnology* 14: 347–56.

———. 1981. Noman: representations of identity in Mount Hagen. In *The Structure of Folk Models,* ed. M. Stuchlik, 281–303. ASA monograph no. 20. London: Academic Press.

———. 1982. Witchcraft, greed, cannibalism and death. In *Death and the Regen-
eration of Life,* ed. Maurice Bloch and J. Parry, 111–133. Cambridge: Cambridge University Press.

———. 1984. *A Line of Power.* London: Tavistock.

———. 1993a. Organs and emotions: the question of metaphor. *Canberra
Anthropology,* 16(2): 1–16.

———. 1993b. *Ru: Biography of a Western Highlander.* Port Moresby, Papua New
Guinea. National Research Institute.

———. 1994a. Between body and mind: shamans and politics among the Anga,
Baktaman and Gebusi in Papua New Guinea. *Oceania,* 64(4): 288–301.

———. 1994b. Keeping the body in mind. *Social Anthropology,* 2(1): 43–53.

———. N.d. Revenge, identity, and honor. Paper presented at the H. F.
Guggenheim Conference, Princeton, N.J.:, 11–13 November 1994.

Strathern, Andrew J., and A. M. Strathern. 1971. *Self-Decoration in Mount Hagen.*
London: Gerald Duckworth Press.

Strathern, Andrew J., and G. Stürzenhofecker, eds. 1994. *Migration and Transformations: Regional Perspectives on New Guinea.* Pittsburgh: University of
Pittsburgh Press (ASAO monograph 15).

Strathern, Marilyn. 1968. Popokl: the question of morality. *Mankind,* 6: 553–562.

———. 1979. The self in self-decoration. *Oceania,* 49: 241–57.

———. 1988. *The Gender of the Gift: Problems with Women and Problems with Society in Melanesia.* Berkeley: University of California Press.

Strauss, Hermann. 1990. *The Mi-Culture of the Mt. Hagen People.* Ed. G. Stürzenhofecker and A. J. Strathern. Trans. Brian Shields. Ethnology Monographs no. 13. Pittsburgh: University of Pittsburgh.

Stürzenhofecker, Gabriele. 1993. Times enmeshed: gender, space and history among the Duna. Ph.D. diss., University of Pittsburgh.

———. 1995. Sacrificial bodies and the cyclicity of substance. *Journal of the Polynesian Society,* 104(1): 1–18.

Synnott, Anthony. 1993. *The Body Social: Symbolism, Self and Society.* London: Routledge.

Taussig, Michael. 1993. *Mimesis and Alterity: A Particular History of the Senses.* London: Routledge.

Taylor, Charles. 1985. The person. In *The Category of the Person,* ed. M. Carrithers et al., 257–81. Cambridge: Cambridge University Press.

———. 1993. To follow a rule . . . . In *Bourdieu: Critical Perspectives,* ed. Craig Calhoun, Edward LiPuma and Moishe Postone, 45–60. Chicago: University of Chicago Press.

Thomas, Nicholas. 1992. Substantivization and anthropological discourse: the transformation of practices into institutions in neo-traditional Pacific societies. In *History and Tradition in Melanesian Anthropology,* ed. James G. Carrier, 64–85. Berkeley: University of California Press.

Thurnwald, Richard. 1916. *Banaro Society.* American Anthropological Association Memoirs 3(4). Lancaster, Pa.: American Anthropological Society.

Turner, Bryan S. 1992. *Regulating Bodies: Essays in Medical Sociology.* London and New York: Routledge.

Varela, Francisco J., Evan Thompson, and Eleanor Rosch. 1991. *The Embodied Mind: Cognitive Science and Human Experience.* Cambridge, Mass.: MIT Press.

Wagner, Roy. 1967. *The Curse of Souw: Principles of Daribi Clan Definition and Alliance.* Chicago: University of Chicago Press.

———. 1972. *Habu: The Innovation of Meaning in Daribi Religion.* Chicago: University of Chicago Press.

———. 1983. The ends of innocence: conception and seduction among the Daribi of Karimui and the Barok of New Ireland. Special issue, ed. D. Jorgensen. *Mankind,* 14(1): 75–83.

Wallace, Edwin R. 1983. *Freud and Anthropology: A History and Appraisal.* New York: International Universities Press.

Wikan, Unni. 1990. *Managing Turbulent Hearts: A Balinese Formula for Living.* Chicago: University of Chicago Press.

Williams, Michael A. 1989. Divine image—prison of flesh: perceptions of the body in ancient Gnosticism. In *Fragments for a History of the Human Body,* ed. M. Feher, R. Naddaff and N. Tazi, 128–145. New York: ZONE Press.

Winkelman, Michael James. 1990. Shamans and other "magico-religious" healers: a cross-cultural study of their origins, nature, and social transformations. *Ethos* 18: 308–52.

Index

Aeschylus, 54
Agency, 28; agency/substance distinction, 108; and the body, 39; heart soul as manifesting among Temiar, 155
Allen, N., 11
Anatomy, 142, 147–48
Ancient Greece, 43–55
Androgyny, 87
Anesthesia, 148–50
Anger: in ancient Greek thought, 45–46; in Hagen (Melpa) thought, 18, 120, 122, 161; in Huli thought, 126; in Ilongot thought, 51; in Pangia (Wiru) thought, 45; in Temiar, 155; in Yupno thought, 119, 121
Ankave, 71
Aristotle, 3, 12, 44, 55
Assipattle, 95
Atkinson, J. M., 153, 158–59, 162–63
Augustine, Saint, 57
Austin, J. L., 30
Australian Aboriginals, 13

Baktaman, 70–71, 78
Barclay, J. (Edinburgh), 147
Barth, F., 70–71, 78
Baruya, 129
Battaglia, D., 7
Baudinet, M.-J., 59
Baudrillard, J., 62
Bemba, 17
Bettelheim, B., 74
Biersack, A., 68–70, 78–80
Bimin, 82–83, 86–87

Biomedicine, 64, 106; adopted in Papua New Guinea, 134–35; anatomy in, 147; assumptions in, 144–47; development of anesthesia and surgery in, 148–50; patient's body as passive in, 150
Blackburn, J., 101–2
Bloch, M., 28, 138
Blood: among Duna, 134; among Gnau, 115–18; among Huli, 124–27; and lineage, 34; menstrual, 68–79; in sacrifice, 45; in Telefomin ideas, 81–82
Boddy, J., 151, 153, 169–71
Body substances/parts: and consumption of, 88 (Hua); hair, 192; Huli ideas about, 127–30; Melanesian ideas of, 64–96, 108–10; Melpa ideas of, 127–30; the nose, among Huli and Duna, 131; one-sex and two-sex models of, 139; representations of skeletons, 147. *See also* Humoral ideas
Bogaia, 130, 133
Bonnemère, P., 71
Boundaries: and bodily symbolism, 14–16, 65, 90–91; in relation to personhood, 153–76; Ruth Padel on 50–51, 53. *See also* Skin
Bourdieu, P., 10, 23, 25–30, 33–38, 55, 62, 164, 177, 197
Bourguignon, E., 153
Brain, 8
Bride-service, 20
Bridewealth (Yupno), 117, 121